"*Real Kids* is a must read for any parent concerned about their child's eating or weight. In a clear and concise way, Kater tells parents how to help their children navigate this fat-phobic world while learning how to avoid eating and weight problems. The skills she outlines will carry children for the rest of their lives. What an incredible gift for any parent to give their child. Make sure you read this powerful book . . . and put it to use!"
—Karin Kratina, PhD, RD, Clinical Advisory Board, NEDO (National Eating Disorders Organization)

"A valuable tool kit of ideas and activities to help develop strong, healthy body esteem in 'kids' of all ages and sizes . . . Kathy skillfully addresses the issues of body image, eating disorders, nutrition, and childhood obesity. Providing readers a rare opportunity to look at their own beliefs and attitudes around these issues and offering specific steps and actions to take to adjust them as needed . . . This book is a vital resource for professionals and parents in bridging the gap between preventing eating disorders and at the same time addressing the increasing prevalence of obesity in kids. A must read for all of us interested in creating healthy children who love their bodies no matter what size they are!"
—Sarah Stinson, MS, eating disorders therapist and Higher*self* director

"Kathy Kater provides the right ingredients for parents, teachers, and health professionals to encourage and teach positive healthy eating, exercise, and body image to children and teens. Not only does Kathy get to the root of the problem with weightism in our society, she provides resources, skills, and healthy solutions to overcome the issues at hand. Bravo!"
—Susan Crowell, MS, RD, LD, registered dietitian

"I LOVE this book . . . I think that *Real Kids Come in All Sizes* should be required reading for all new parents. I am certain that if this were the case the incidence of obesity and eating disorders would decrease. We need to address these issues and Kathy's book brings insight and understanding to an issue that is very complicated and perplexing for most of us. It gives very practical advice and easy-to-follow sensible lessons."
—Kitty Westin, President, The Anna Westin Foundation

"As an internist who cares for women with eating disorders, and a parent of two elementary-age daughters, I am ecstatic to have a book that gets at the nuts and bolts of body esteem. *Real Kids Come in All Sizes* reads eas-

ily and offers a wealth of information for parents, educators, and health professionals. As a community, if we follow Ms. Kater's curriculum to maintain and nurture healthy body esteem in our children, eating disorders and teen violence could become a thing of the past."
—Sonia Kragh, MD, Syracuse, NY

"As a registered dietitian I have worked with many clients who suffer from a negative body image. This long overdue book is an invaluable resource for parents to help their children develop and maintain strong body esteem and a healthy body image. The author provides sensible and practical advice on motivating children to eat well for health and well-being, and not to achieve an unrealistic body size. Bravo!"
—Janice Newell Bissex, MS, RD, author of *The Moms' Guide to Meal Makeovers*

"Given our national preoccupation with perfect bodies, this book is an important guide for concerned parents who want to build healthy self-acceptance in their children."
—Joan Jacobs Brumberg, author of *The Body Project: An Intimate History of American Girls* and *Fasting Girls: The History of Anorexia Nervosa*

"Through her workshops and curriculum, Kathy Kater has effectively gotten kids and families in touch with reality about body image. Now, anyone anywhere can tap her powerful, easy-to-understand concepts. *Real Kids Come in All Sizes* is an essential tool for adults who care about kids in our marketing-saturated and appearance-first culture. We can fight for our children's souls and win!"
—Joe Kelly, President, Dads and Daughters®, and author of *Dads and Daughters: How to Inspire, Support, and Understand Your Daughter* (Broadway, 2003)

"Kathy Kater's *Healthy Body Image* (HBI) curriculum is a wonderful program, and the Board of Jewish Education has urged its use in elementary schools. For many students, these are their 'favorite classes' and parents are heartened that their children are learning these important lessons so enthusiastically. *Real Kids Come in All Sizes* is the perfect supplement to the HBI curriculum, as now parents can be educated in how to support the curriculum concepts, and most importantly, how to help their children be healthy and feel comfortable with their bodies."
—Shayna Oppen, CSW, Director, Dept. of Student Health Services, Board of Jewish Education of Greater New York

REAL KIDS COME IN ALL SIZES

REAL KIDS COME IN ALL SIZES

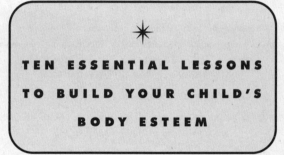

TEN ESSENTIAL LESSONS TO BUILD YOUR CHILD'S BODY ESTEEM

KATHY KATER

A LARK PRODUCTION

BROADWAY BOOKS

NEW YORK

PRINTED IN THE UNITED STATES OF AMERICA

BROADWAY BOOKS and its logo, a letter B bisected on the diagonal,
are trademarks of Random House, Inc.

Visit our website at www.broadwaybooks.com

First edition published 2004

Book design by Chris Welch
Illustrated by Andrew Barthelmes

Library of Congress Cataloging-in-Publication Data
Kater, Kathy.
Real kids come in all sizes : ten essential lessons to build your
child's body esteem / Kathy Kater.
p.   cm.
1. Body image in children.   2. Self-esteem in children.
3. Child rearing.   I. Title.

BF723.B6K38 2004
649'.1—dc22

2003064628

ISBN 0-7679-1608-5

1   3   5   7   9   10   8   6   4   2

ACKNOWLEDGMENTS

The National Eating Disorder Association published my *Healthy Body Image: Teaching Kids to Eat and Love Their Bodies Too!* prevention curriculum for upper elementary age kids in 1998. The positive response from educators and parents was the catalyst for this book, and it seems fitting that my first words of appreciation go to NEDA for their support. Even more, however, I am indebted to the more than five hundred clients who trusted me with their stories of conflict and pain in bodies they learned to feel far too at odds with. I hope all of you take heart in knowing that what I have learned from you may help the next generation of children find an easier, healthier path.

Through this entire project, my husband Lincoln's constant belief that my work can make a difference, his endless support, patience, editing, and willingness to constantly reassure me in insecure moments served as my rock. I cannot thank him enough for making my efforts possible. My daughter Anya's constant challenges required me to dig deep for my best self, while my son Adam's pride in his mom's work eased the way. Both gave me the energy as well as a sense of purpose and strength to get the job done. Likewise, I want to thank my three sisters, Julie, Caroline, and Jackie, for still being there through the years of neglect when I have given my all to this work.

To my friends who told me again and again they expected to see me on *Oprah* one day, please know how grateful I am for your support. To Joe Kelly, of Dads and Daughters, I am indebted for the inspiration you provided, for the vision and passion we share, and for your bear hugs. Also for sending me to Robin Dellabough at Lark Productions, who did all you promised she would in securing a great publisher for this book, as well as providing the expertise to put it together. I am grateful that Trish Medved saw the book's potential early on and championed it from start to finish. She and her able assistant, Beth Datlowe, also provided terrific editorial help along the way.

I am indebted as well to many colleagues who are working tirelessly in this uphill battle to prevent and treat body image, eating, and weight problems in our culture. I would like to single out Dr. Michael P. Levine, who, in addition to being a brilliant academician and researcher in the area of eating disorder prevention, is an amazing, selflessly driven human being who steered me in the right direction from the start and gave me confidence to move out of the safety of my clinical practice into the arena of prevention. Finally, thank you to all who have written to tell me that my curriculum or workshops have made a difference in your life. Please know that you too have made a difference through your support.

CONTENTS

FOREWORD

✳

M edical science continues to amaze us with major break-
throughs in technology, new antibiotics, heroic surgical maneuvers, and growing understanding of the
genetic code. In the face of these miraculous discoveries, it is
easy to forget the basic building blocks for health and well-
being: healthy body image and body esteem, balanced eating
habits and choices, and regular exercise.

As a pediatrician, I know that prevention is key, whether we
consider immunizations for diphtheria or polio, screening every
newborn for hearing impairment, or discussing safe sexual
practices with young adolescents. By providing these simple,
relatively inexpensive interventions early on, we have found we
can effectively avoid many destructive or unhappy outcomes.
When we look far upstream from the visible disorders of obesity, anorexia nervosa, and bulimia we see the insidious,
contributory seeds of body dissatisfaction, poor self-esteem, restrictive and inappropriate food choices, and lack of exercise.
Addressing these less tangible problems through early inter-

vention is a prevention initiative that we desperately need today.

Practicing medicine in a busy urban county hospital, I see many patients who present me with challenges affecting their health and well-being. I frequently encounter children and adolescents whose problems stem from negative body images and dangerous diet and exercise practices. Almost daily, I ponder the best approach to treating children and teens weighing over 250 or 300 pounds with hip problems, type II diabetes, social isolation, and, on the other end of the spectrum, lovely young girls engaging in restrictive diets or over-the-counter diet aids to shed pounds and inches. By the time these end-stage problems surface, the window of opportunity for full recovery is closing. In *Real Kids Come in All Sizes*, Kathy Kater draws from twenty-five years of clinical experience, as well as from the latest research, to provide an approach that teaches parents to intervene before destructive attitudes and habits have a chance to grow. Helping us to see that these disorders share many common root causes, we see that teaching children positive attitudes and healthy alternatives at an early age is our greatest hope of prevention.

I am privileged to care for teens from dozens of countries around the world, as well as those who are American-born from a variety of cultural and ethnic backgrounds. Increasingly, even recent young immigrants to America are caught up in a frenzy of dieting to lose weight: "I am too fat"; "My mother thinks I am too big"; "I want to look like an American." Ironically, many of these teens come from countries where famine and hunger are rife. Kathy Kater makes the elegant and vitally important point in *Real Kids Come in All*

Sizes about genetic potential and biological destiny. The general height and weight expected for a child or teen depend on many unalterable factors. Cultural pressures urging conformity to an unrealistic idealized image in order to fit in are dangerous and inappropriate. Children, teens, and parents who face the challenge of assimilation into American culture need to hear congruent messages that promote health and healthy lifestyle choices at all sizes and shapes. But even American parents often have trouble resisting unhealthy pressures about weight and eating. When my own four children, now adolescents and young adults, navigated minefields of harmful media images and societal expectations, my husband and I often felt uncertain about the right advice to impart, let alone the most effective role-modeling. In this book, parents will find important background information that reviews and debunks the cultural myths about thinness and dieting. In Part II, ten lessons provide parents with helpful information and suggestions to encourage positive body esteem, healthy eating practices, and fitness in their children.

Even as I praise this innovative book and feel confident that parents (and teachers and physicians, as well) will find the information useful and accessible, we must all keep certain barriers in mind. Too often the nutritionally dense foods children need are expensive and complex to prepare for families struggling with low income and isolation. Many children living in unsafe neighborhoods do not and cannot enjoy daily recreation and exercise. With funding cuts, schools have decreased the number of physical education hours, and health club membership is not possible for many with limited budgets. Communities, governmental agencies, and car-

ing adults have a responsibility to ensure that recommendations for healthy lifestyles through good nutrition and physical activity are options that are available for *all* children.

Marjorie J. Hogan, M.D., pediatrician
Pediatrics and Adolescent Medicine, Hennepin County
  Medical Center
Director of Pediatric Medical Education, HCMC
Associate Professor of Pediatrics, University of Min-
  nesota

PROLOGUE

GRASS WON'T GROW THERE

This story is a gift from a woman I'll call JoAnn. While the specifics of JoAnn's life are uniquely her own, the struggle with her body is virtually that of Everywoman since the 1960s. Change a few details, and you will find yourself or someone you know.

JoAnn was petite, muscular, and lean through her early forties. Then, with no change in her eating or her lifestyle of jogging, hiking, skiing, in-line skating, and biking, her midlife body began to take on a different shape. In particular, a layer of fat was added that no amount of exercise would eliminate. In the past ten years JoAnn has struggled daily against the weight her middle-aged body wants to be.

Although still strong and fit, JoAnn hated the appearance of her softer shape. She stopped listening to her normal hunger and began to diet. At first she dropped pounds, but inevitably they would return when her restricted hunger broke free and demanded satisfaction. The more she dieted, the more her food cravings seemed to take control, and she would consume all the calories she had avoided and more. After five years of dieting, an increased self-loathing, and twenty extra pounds, she was obsessed with food. Although terrified that if she ate, she would not be able to stop, she started to binge on sweets, especially chocolate. In true and typical form, the more JoAnn tried to avoid food, the more consumed she became with it. On her fiftieth birthday, thirty pounds fatter than her five-foot-two-inch body had ever been, she was diagnosed with an eating disorder.

Sometime during the ten years in which her eating disorder was germinating, JoAnn developed an interest in gardening. Was there a connection between her devotion to *stopping* the growth of her body size and *starting* new growth in her yard? Most of JoAnn's yard was responsive to what she planted, but one area in particular plagued her—a sunless strip near her back fence, overshadowed by her neighbor's large, dense trees and bushes. In the early years that JoAnn had lived in her home, this foliage had not been so tall, and an uninterrupted expanse of lush grass had run all the way back to the fence. But the conditions had changed, and in the dense shade, the grass had grown thinner year by year. This was *not* JoAnn's vision for her yard. In an effort to renew the grass she had previously loved, JoAnn spent six or seven summers repeatedly seeding new grass, fertilizing, watering, and all but singing lullabies to the shaded earth. A promising flush of velvety green sprouts would appear each May, only to become thin, weak blades groping for the sun by August. When the snow melted the following spring, the expanse of bare and brown ground would reappear along her back fence.

The more JoAnn heard the advice that grass would not grow in the shade, the more determined she became. She would set her jaw, buy more seed, and look for other reasons for the failure of her grass. Each spring, a new crop of hopeful, germinated seedlings seduced JoAnn. She would call to her neighbors, "Come and look at my grass! It's beautiful; just the way I want it." It didn't seem fair that the seeds should sprout so well and give so much hope, if by August they could not be maintained.

Last year JoAnn went into treatment for her eating disorder. Despite the therapy, she has not yet been able to feel safe satisfying her hunger or allowing her body to assume its natural weight at this stage of her life. But last spring, when she looked out at her bare, shaded dirt JoAnn fought with her instinct to try again with the grass. For the last time, she painfully turned the soil and covered the few wisps of grass that still stood. In the space along her fence she planted thirty-five shade-loving hosta plants, laced intermittently with delicate, woodland ferns.

The new plants quickly took root and began to grow lush and green in their natural element, cool and hidden from the sun, creating a rich, thick border between the bright grassy yard and the fence. This spring JoAnn's call to her neighbors contained the same joy, "Come look at my beautiful, green yard!" When July turned to August, the new plants still filled the space with an attractive mass of foliage.

Could this newfound understanding of the limits of her lawn and appreciation of another form of beauty encourage JoAnn's acceptance of her body's natural limits? Such changes in body image are not so simple. JoAnn still fights and fails daily to defy her biology. Making peace with her body and moving on to a new image for herself will probably be a longer, tougher road than the seven or eight years it took JoAnn to accept a new look for her yard.

In my clinical practice I have many clients like JoAnn who have been fighting the same battle of their bodies since they were young teens. While JoAnn was lucky to have avoided years of misery in her earlier life, she is the exception in that regard. Body image and eating problems do not easily disappear as we grow up. Far better to help our children avoid this path and resist the myths that encourage it from the start.

INTRODUCTION

✳

J ust before entering fourth grade, my daughter asked me why her best friend would call herself "fat." While playing one day, her friend apparently announced that because she was fat she could no longer eat peanut butter and could only have one piece of bread in her sandwich. She also drank diet soda instead of milk. My daughter was confused. First, she couldn't really see the fatness her friend was talking about— because it wasn't there. Furthermore, the idea of deciding how much to eat based on real or imagined *fatness* rather than on satisfying one's hunger sounded very strange to her.

As a psychotherapist who had treated body image, eating, and weight disorders for more than twenty years, I knew only too well where my daughter's friend was coming from. At the age of nine, these previously happy, unself-conscious girls were about to enter puberty in the context of a culture where their chances to feel good about their bodies and be comfortable with their appetites were marginal. I was not surprised by this reality, but neither was I ready for my own daughter to be exposed to it.

Each client I meet in my clinical practice brings hope for her own recovery. But it's discouraging that there is still no end in sight to the stream of new and increasingly young victims. Despite the progress that has been made in understanding the causes and treating the symptoms of body image, eating, and weight concerns (the primary risk factors for eating disorders), this new awareness has not yet led to effective prevention. Instead, these problems have become more common—so common that it is currently abnormal if an adolescent American girl feels good about her body. Boys are increasingly affected as well. It is extremely difficult to change negative body esteem and eating behaviors once they are established, and the cost in health, self-confidence, quality of life, and dollars is just too great. It's time to stop these problems before they start—beginning with our children. The good news is that we now know how to do just that, if enough adults understand the issues and take on the challenge.

The most common body-image complaint is "feeling fat." Notice that *feeling* fat is not the same thing as *being* fat. Feeling fat is a uniquely Western concept. It arises from the subjective, self-critical conviction that part or all of a person's body is fatter than it "should" be according to an idealized standard. Believe it or not, it is quite possible to be fat without this self-condemnation. A five-foot-six, two-hundred-pound woman in a non-Western culture might not feel fat, while most females of *any* size and shape in the United States do.

The so-called solution for feeling fat is dieting to lose weight. Dieting has become a normal eating style in the United States, even among healthy-weight individuals. Given our concern that America has now become the fattest nation on earth, you may wonder, "What's wrong with that?" What's wrong is that the attitudes and reasoning that lead to feeling fat and rampant dieting are fatally flawed. In fact, dieting has added to the unhealthy fattening of our population. Dieting routinely leads to habits that swing from inadequate, restrictive eating one day to excessive high-calorie binges the next. Rather than helping, this "solution" has become part of the problem. In the same four decades during which America's drive to be thin has produced the greatest weight-loss efforts ever known to humankind, America has simultaneously become the fattest nation on earth! The slimmer we have tried to be, the fatter we have become. Typical eating habits in the land of plenty are among the worst in the world.

We already know that the self-esteem of American girls drops dramatically with the onset of puberty. Major contributing factors to this decrease are our culture's nonstop, harshly judgmental body scrutiny, intense fear of fatness, and pervasive belief in the need to deny hunger to avoid body loathing. The United States is the only country in the world in which the natural rounding out of a girl's body in puberty triggers the statistical probability of body disdain and a lowered sense of self-esteem. This means that simultaneous with their budding independence and unfolding womanhood, our girls develop a dangerous psychological vulnerability. This vulnerability leads girls to think it's worth sacrificing their nutritional needs in hopes of achieving, regaining, or maintaining the right body. As if this is not bad enough, the time and energy girls forfeit worrying about whether they look fat, scrutinizing their silhouettes in every window and mirror, and in general feeling bad in their own skin is beyond measure. Feeling fat and the unhealthy eating that accompanies it are disturbing, plain and simple, and put victims at risk for a host of more serious problems as well. Thanks to the cultural factors that have created this situation, by age twelve roughly half of all American girls will relate to this statement by a twenty-two-year-old in recovery from bulimia:

Actually I felt pretty good about my body until about sixth grade. But then everyone else hated theirs, so I thought I should too.

By age fourteen, two-thirds will feel this way:

Why should I eat healthy if it won't make me thin?

Words like these are a call to arms for parents: preventing the erosion of body esteem in girls and boys is not a luxury. We cannot wait to take serious action.

Not long after my fourth-grade daughter's question about her fat-fearing friend, I had an epiphany. I knew that my clients often struggle for months and even years to accept the essential lessons needed to recover from their unhealthy body image and eating problems. It dawned on me that these same basic lessons about body size and shape are elementary enough for a fourth-grade child to understand—without having to first undo all the weightist, thin-ideal mumbo jumbo. Soon after, I began the intensive research that led to a new, comprehensive prevention curriculum for upper-elementary schoolchildren. Called *Healthy Body Image: Teaching Kids to Eat and Love Their Bodies Too!*, its goals were simple but revolutionary in America today:

1. To help children maintain a healthy relationship to the bodies with which they were born.
2. To motivate children to eat well and be active for the sake

of health, fitness, satisfaction, and well-being—not in an effort to manipulate body size.

Several years of classroom testing has shown that the *Healthy Body Image* curriculum lessons are effective. Results demonstrate that when we get the right messages to children early enough, we can make a significant positive difference. The information in my curriculum gives children knowledge, tools, and realistic attitudes with which to resist unhealthy cultural pressures about body image. Now *Real Kids Come in All Sizes* offers this vital information to parents, showing you how to integrate body-esteem building concepts into your everyday life with your children. Part 1 provides background information that is necessary to understand the body-image pressures your child faces today. Part 2 offers ten essential lessons to help your child maintain strong body esteem and healthy body image.

BEFORE YOU BEGIN

It's important to understand that this book is not about the prevention of eating disorders, although it is intended to prevent many of the *conditions* that put kids at risk for these life-threatening problems. (A reading list in appendix D will help you find additional information on this topic.) The primary risk factors known to trigger eating disorders are (1) feeling fat, and (2) the belief that dieting is an effective weight-loss strategy. The two factors exist in the midrange of a continuum that ranges from healthy body image and eating on one end, through varying degrees of body dissatisfaction and unwholesome eating, to diagnosable eating disorders on the other. (See appendix A on page 229 for a self-evaluation of where you fall on the continuum.) While eating disorders are extremely serious, the number of children for whom these disorders will be triggered is still relatively small. On the other hand, the vast majority of people today, especially girls, will struggle with negative body image and poor eating habits. I frankly assume that many of you have your own body-image demons and are as caught up as everyone else in the American weight mythology. But whether or not you battle your body size, you can help your child resist recruitment for this lifelong conflict. In this book I try to guide all parents to help all children maintain the body esteem they were born with. I fully expect the lessons I share will be useful tools in the prevention of eating disorders as well.

WHAT ARE HEALTHY BODY IMAGE AND POSITIVE BODY ESTEEM?

Negative body image has become familiar to so many people that *healthy* body image and esteem sound almost foreign. We have to understand their meanings and how they are different to achieve our goals.

Body image: The outside view

Body image includes our mental picture of how we look from the outside, along with our thoughts and feelings *about* that picture. You may be surprised to know that body image, in and of itself, does not start out as positive or negative. While small children are often curious about how they look, they do not usually judge their appearance one way or the other. For example, a small child might see a red-haired girl with braids, green eyes, freckles, a rounded tummy, and dimpled knees in the mirror—but will not evaluate this look as good or bad.

Placing a value on what we see in the mirror is something we learn to do as a result of several factors—some real, and some made up from experiences we have had and stories we have learned to believe about looks. Feelings about our body's appearance are swayed by events that draw attention to our body: illness, trauma, surgery, or normal developmental changes (such as puberty), as well as our own innate aesthetic preferences (we may be more drawn to blue eyes than green). In addition, exposure to messages that clearly value one way to look over another begin to have a cumulative effect.

As body image takes on value, a child begins to see that to be taller or shorter, fatter or thinner is no longer simply a fact, but may be judged positively or negatively. If, for example, people compliment red hair and green eyes, but point and laugh at a rounded tummy and dimpled knees, an insecurity that didn't previously exist may arise: "Are my looks OK?" Suddenly, how we think we look from the outside takes on a new importance and includes a sense of vulnerability. You may not have realized that an evaluation of looks creates vulnerability regardless of whether the judgment is "good" or "bad," since this places the power for acceptability in the hands of someone else. *How much* vulnerability can depend on many factors, such as a child's sensitivity to outside criticism, her personality type, the degree to which her body fits the cultural "ideal," the nature, frequency, and intensity of body messages a child is exposed to, and the context in which those messages are sent.

Many variables that may affect body image are *not in a parent's control*. There are two important things we can do to help our children resist negative influences, however. In ad-

dition to teaching kids to question and critically assess messages from the outside world that evaluate body appearance,
we can help them combat unrealistic and unhealthy messages by reinforcing their innate *body esteem*.

Body esteem: The inside view

Have you ever tried to feed a baby who was not hungry or to
lay one down when it wanted to be held? If so, you have witnessed the purest form of positive body esteem. Newborns
and toddlers do not need outside cues to tell them what they
feel. They are connected to their own inner experience, have
no doubt about its validity, and confidently use their voices to
express this day or night. From the inside out, babies demonstrate healthy body esteem: they trust their senses, independent of external cues about how they *should* be feeling or
what we think they should want. The essence of body esteem
at any age is to be in touch with and positively regard our inner experience without doubt or judgment. Thoughts *about*
or judgments *of* this reality may be important to consider, but
these are nonetheless secondary. What is primary is a secure
sense of "knowing" our inner experience. The most notable
aspect of positive body esteem is that, whether or not the outside world agrees, we are the ultimate authority. We are "in"
our body.

Healthy body esteem does not sacrifice the confident
"knowing" of our own experience even as we tune in to others. Whether we are hungry or full, energetic or tired, prefer
oranges or grapes—we know this is true for us even if no one
else feels the same and even if what we need isn't obtainable.
Healthy body esteem means maintaining integrity: we know
what we need, even when circumstances do not support us.

Reinforcing body esteem in our children means helping them to stay connected to and maintain trust in themselves even when this trust is challenged. For example, one night while eating dinner at his grandparent's home, my then eight-year-old son's grandfather—a well-intentioned, but gruff, authoritarian man—urged a serving of creamed onions on him. To my son's polite, "No, thank you. I don't care for onions," came his grandfather's righteous roar, "You don't know what you like!" Fortunately my husband was present and diffused his father's wrath while firmly validating our son's ability to know his own tastes. The important lesson was to affirm that our son should not disconnect from the truth of his own experience to avoid displeasing his grandfather. While it's unlikely this was a pivotal moment in our son's life, life is made up of thousands of such events, including some situations that are much more seriously compromising. Fat children are told all the time that they "can't be hungry!" Slim, "beautiful" children are told that they "can't be sad or lonely!" Such discountings are lessons in disconnection.

If frequent messages that contradict what children know to be true go unchallenged or unexplained by adults, underlying trust in who they are (and therefore their body esteem) begins to break down. People who are unhappy with their bodies share several traits that reflect a breakdown of body esteem. They are not sure what they feel, at least in some areas of their life. It is hard for them to trust the inner voice that tells them what they want and don't want independent of what *others* may want for them or expect of them. Their description of self is often based on what they believe or fear others may think about them, particularly when it comes to how they look, since this aspect of self can't really be hidden.

They worry that they may want or need too much for others to tolerate. Since eating demonstrates a need, they fear their hunger and appetite may be too big or (rarely) too small. What if they take up too much space or time in a way that others don't like? At the same time, they worry they won't be "enough." They fear others won't approve. People who are unhappy with their bodies often believe they must *tune out* from what is true for them in order to tune in to what they believe others want from them.

If you recognize some of these tendencies, you're not unusual. This externalization of self is common, perhaps increasingly common in today's world in which we are routinely bombarded day after day by advertising propaganda telling us what we should want and who we should be in order to be desirable to others. Since the wish to be desirable and included is universal, we are all susceptible to erosion of body esteem *if we can be convinced to believe this sacrifice is necessary to stay connected to others.*

Healthy body esteem is extremely important in becoming an independent, healthy person in general. This is all the more true in a cultural context that systematically teaches children to sacrifice trust in their body in order to be included. When we find growing numbers of girls and boys (like my daughter's nine-year-old friend) who feel they must restrict their natural appetites, who mistrust the cues that will let them know when they are hungry and full, and who fear their bodies will betray them, we see the alarming outcome of the breakdown of body esteem. Rather than trusting themselves to unfold from the inside out, living up to their potential through wholesome eating and physical activity, America's children are learning to think of their bodies as disconnected packages they should manipulate externally for the "right" appearance or entertain with the latest high-calorie treat. If messages that erode healthy body esteem go unchallenged, reliance on external standards that objectify bodies will increase your child's risk for unhealthy body image and eating. On the other hand, when messages that reinforce healthy body esteem are provided at an early age, children will be less likely to disconnect from what they really need for health and well-being.

We are still learning what it will take to help kids maintain positive self-esteem as they move through the critical middle school and high school years. Without a doubt, this is an uphill battle that flies in the face of pressures that demand that we ignore our authentic selves as we strive for unrealistic "ideals." One thing is clear: success depends on active adult participation. This requires learning how to effectively challenge the pervasive messages that blatantly support negative body-image attitudes and unhealthy eating.

A popular saying suggests that for a cultural problem to be perpetuated, all it takes is for enlightened people to do nothing. There are many harsh or dangerous factors that may affect our children over which we have no control and may not be able to do anything about. This is no longer true when it comes to arming our children to resist negative body-image messages and eating habits. We now know enough to prevent children from falling prey to the unquestioned belief that how they look is more important than who they are. The right messages can stop children from berating themselves for not having the right body, from sacrificing their energy and nutritional needs in no-win attempts to reshape their biological destiny, and as a result, from compromising their health and emotional well-being.

Real Kids Come in All Sizes will guide you and, in turn,

your children to a more nourishing and nurturing alternative. Together we can help the next generation of children value themselves and each other, not based on the size of their clothes or the shape of their thighs, but based on the unique qualities of their character, talent, ability, friendship, and humanity.

Note to reader: Although I wrote this book for parents of both boys and girls, for simplicity's sake—and because far more girls are affected by body-image concerns than boys—I've used the female pronoun in most instances. Also, throughout this book, unless otherwise specified, the words diet *and* dieting *should be defined in the following way: restricted eating according to an external plan that prescribes not only what but how much to eat for the purpose of losing weight.*

PART ONE

✳

CHAPTER 1

BODY IMAGE BLUES

Sounding the Alarm

Too many American children, particularly girls, are afraid to gain weight. The compelling wish to be thin or stay thin at all costs provides the seeds for a lifetime of intense, unrelenting, counterproductive conflict between hunger and eating, or between the body they were born with and, as diet advertisements promise, "the body you always wanted." Ironically, hand in hand with the greatest weight-loss campaign ever known, an epidemic number of Americans have become unhealthily fat.

It is startling to recognize that this conflicted way of relating to our bodies is now the norm in our country. But the outrage of our shock may drain into resignation when we realize just how big this problem has become. After all, what can we do if so many people battle their bodies? My goal is to make you believe there is plenty we can do. The house is burning, but we now know enough about the fuel that is feeding this fire to put it out—if we take action together. First, let's sound the alarm.

BEAUTY AND THE BODY

Between 65 and 85 percent of adult women in the United States *do not* feel good about their bodies. Many men are affected as well. Most say this is because they are or *feel* fat, which may or may not reflect *being* fat. This dissatisfaction is not trivial. Surveys show that a lot of women would trade several years of life and career success for the opportunity to permanently lose fifteen to twenty pounds. Most of these unhappy individuals routinely engage in unhealthy dieting that in turn leaves them obsessed with food and ashamed of their hunger.

By the time they are in eighth grade, roughly 75 percent of our still-growing girls have adopted this distrust of and bad feelings about their bodies and have learned that they too should try to take control of the matter by dieting. At a time in their lives when they should feel secure in their body's growth, developing confidence in habits that would help them to become healthy adults with diverse, healthy weights, American children are increasingly worried about size. Kids who should be focusing on tasks that will help them grow intellectually, emotionally, artistically, socially, and physically are instead distracted and anxious about weight. Mothers feel helpless to intervene, fearful their daughters may be excluded for being too large. Fathers do not know what to say when their naturally rounding pubescent girls ask, "Am I fat?"

We see the toll of poor body image on younger and younger children. Once thought of as an adolescent problem, now almost half of normal weight third- to sixth-grade girls say they would "like to lose weight," and up to one-third say they have already tried dieting. We have not taught these kids to feel integrity in their bodies, nor that we want them to eat well for health and well-being. Instead, from a very early age they have learned to feel there is something wrong with them. Girls from the richest country in the world have been raised to worry first and foremost that they are not the size or shape they have come to believe they should be and that they cannot trust their natural hunger.

BODY-IMAGE MESSAGES

How often do you:

- Talk about feeling fat?
- Say you should go on a diet or talk about being on a weight-loss diet?
- Bemoan that you have gone off your diet and that you have eaten "too much"—again!
- Imply you were "bad" for eating something?
- Speak negatively about one or more body parts (e.g., "I hate my thighs!")?
- Make fun of or criticize people's size or shape?
- Comment negatively about how much people eat?

MALE BODY-IMAGE WORRIES

Boys are not immune to body-image concerns, although only a handful of studies have measured how boys and men feel about their bodies. Perhaps this is because the number of males who develop a diagnosable eating disorder is small. Fewer than 1 percent of men are diagnosed with these debilitating disorders, compared to between 5 and 10 percent of girls. The difference is even greater for partial-syndrome eating disorders (in which several, but not all of the criteria for a full-blown, diagnosable eating disorder are met). Estimates suggest that 30 percent of postpubescent females have partial-syndrome eating disorders, compared to only 2 percent of males.

Nonetheless, body dissatisfaction in males is on the increase. For most boys, the appearance of body fat is cause for some unhappiness, but it is the rise in their desire for a "ripped" (highly muscular) look that has drawn the most attention. For example, in 1972, only 18 percent of males said they "disliked their upper torso," but by 2004 the percentage had risen to between 45 and 55 percent.

While few studies exist, there is consensus that males have been affected by a significant rise in the number of images of "ideal" pumped-up men in today's mass media. A recent cover of *Men's Health* magazine offers an example of the standard that men are now challenged to achieve:

> *"Get the abs that drive women wild. Only four weeks to be the trim, muscular guy you've always known you could be!"*

The heightened focus on bodybuilding, excessive musculature, and unnatural leanness is less motivated by health than by a growing insecurity about appearance in boys and men. Bodybuilding as a sport has been around for some time, but an increase in compulsive weightlifting and consumption of bulking-up substances has clearly gone hand in hand with changes in media images of men. We've also seen a rise in products that can be purchased to supposedly achieve the "ideal" male look. Most alarming is the increase—even among boys of middle school age—in use of anabolic steroids to build muscles and exaggerate male sexual characteristics.

While these drugs are not legal without a prescription, abusers find ways to obtain them, and advice about their use is readily available on the Internet. The effectiveness of these drugs makes them extremely seductive, and most users are either not aware of or deny the serious medical complications that are inevitable with long-term use.

G.I. JOE BULKS UP

A study published in *The International Journal of Eating Disorders* made the news by reporting curious changes in G.I. Joe, Luke Skywalker, Batman, and several other male action figures over the past thirty years. Findings show that if G.I. Joe was life-size, between 1973 and 1998 his chest would have increased from 44.4 inches to 54.8 inches and his biceps from 12.2 inches to 26.8 inches. The authors noted that, "G.I. Joe now sports larger biceps than any bodybuilder in history." Although his waist increased also (from 31.7 inches to 36.5 inches) he has "the sharply rippled abdominals of an advanced bodybuilder," whereas the early models have far less definition.

Although boys are now pressured into body-image worry along with girls, boys for the most part channel their concerns differently than girls. Boys who feel bad about their bodies are more likely than girls to divert their feelings into external things, such as sports, music, cars, and academics. They learn to use tools to build engines or empires outside of themselves. This focus on external projects that can be accomplished with their bodies may help many boys keep appearance concerns in check.

GIRLS INTERNALIZE PROBLEMS

Girls, on the other hand, do the opposite. Girls direct their body-image concerns inward and make their bodies into a project. Joan Blomberg's book *The Body Project* demonstrates how much time, attention, money, and self-esteem girls spend working on transforming and reshaping their natural endowment. By studying the diaries of girls and women, Blomberg found that a shift has occurred in values and attitudes over the past one hundred years. From their writings we see that women have always been interested in physical attractiveness: longing for a new dress for the dance, wondering whether to encourage or discourage the natural bend or straightness of hair, what color to paint lips, and at what age to begin. But in the first half of the twentieth century, diary entries regularly reflected the common value of the community: character was held as more important than beauty. Early-twentieth-century girls who wished for good looks soon refocused their concern to emphasize *good works*—a humble wish to be a better person—or at least to project attractiveness by demonstrating deeper qualities, such as honesty, thoughtfulness, generosity, intelligence, humor, and a willingness to work hard.

In contrast, during the last half of the twentieth century, the diary entries of girls changed radically. Gone is the balance of concern between external and internal beauty. This equilibrium is overrun by worry about what shows on the surface. Girls' diaries reflect the preoccupied and anxious belief that outer beauty is paramount. Self-improvement has taken on a different focus entirely. Writings assume an increasingly frantic tone.

In my own work I've often seen the journal entries of clients confirming this urgent, narrow focus:

> *I wish…, I need…, I HAVE to lose 5 pounds by the dance,… 20 pounds by the wedding,… 40 pounds by summer,… or I'd rather die!*

Or as a gorgeous-by-any-standard five-foot-four-inch, 115-pound eighth grader told me: "I hate my body. I am an ugly, fat freak! I know you don't believe this, but really, looks are everything in school. If I don't lose ten pounds this summer, I might as well not even go to high school."

With heightened concern about external presentation, today's females too often abandon the goal of becoming a more engaging and contributing person. We cannot help but worry about pressures that encourage self-centered insecurity about appearance when studies tell us that one of the best predictors of happiness is an altruistic sense of purpose outside ourselves.

Many people believe that unless body image and eating concerns progress to an eating disorder, there is no reason to be so worried. And since only a small percentage of kids develop eating disorders, it can't be all that bad. But how kids feel in their own skins is not trivial, either to them or to the culture at large. There are four major ways that body-image concerns cost our children, our families, and our society at large.

THE COST OF BODY-IMAGE CONCERNS

1. Time, attention, energy, self-esteem, and money drain

At the very least, the mental and emotional drain caused by body dissatisfaction is a huge and painful distraction, consuming a tremendous amount of energy and attention that kids need for more important developmental tasks. Body self-consciousness feels bad, provokes feelings of shame, erodes self-esteem, and makes it very difficult, if not impossible, to concentrate. Kids who routinely worry about their size and shape as they walk down hallways or sit at their desks are anxious and preoccupied students. Kids who feel they are being watched as they eat (or don't eat!) in lunchrooms or who worry about how they look while dressing for or participating in physical education feel awful. Body self-consciousness hampers children's ability to focus on academic, social, daily-living, and other important life skills.

2. A crisis of disconnection

Children with poor body image learn to view themselves from the outside in, rather than the inside out. "How I look" becomes more important than "who I am." As a psychotherapist charged with helping people find their true selves, I can tell you this is a very troubling psychological stance—the antithesis of healthy body esteem, in which the goal is to stay connected to what we know as a guide for healthy development.

As teachers across the country try to guide students to find their voice, to write from their hearts, and to think independently, our culture's focus on external appearance provides a counterattack. Mary Pipher's eloquent book *Reviving Ophelia* caused an intense response in 1994 when she wrote about the ways in which girls today are taught to discount, dissociate, and detach from who they are inside. Her book is just as relevant a decade later. Noted psychologist and eating-disorder treatment specialist Catherine Steiner-Adair, Ed.D., writes:

> *Adolescent girls experience a split between the "me" who presents to the world her best guess of what will be favorably received, and the "real me" who often does not fit the cultural definition of acceptability. Children begin earlier and earlier to expend a lot of effort trying to guess what that externally defined "right" way to look, think, or feel is, and to hide what is often their true selves both from themselves and from others. Self-worth is laid at the mercy of the latest fad and the judgment of the crowd, based on the most superficial of qualities over which we have remarkably little control.*

3. Poor nutrition and spiraling fatness

Negative body image is the number one risk factor for many of the nutrient-deficient, counterproductive, unhealthy, and disordered eating habits that are now routine for many Americans. Instead of being guided by knowledge of good nutrition and natural hunger, eating or not eating is used either to achieve a particular body size or to console ourselves when we fail. While "normal dieting" does not qualify as an eating disorder, eating habits that disregard the primary purpose of eating for nutritional sustenance and satisfaction of hunger are a type of Russian roulette with Mother Nature, jeopardizing the work of the internal weight regulatory system. As a result, many if not most Americans swing from restrictive eating one day to overloads the next, no longer in touch with what it means to eat normally, and often adding pounds along the way.

4. Eating disorders

Last, body-image concerns can lead to life-threatening, developmentally disruptive, energy-draining, and difficult-to-treat eating disorders such as anorexia nervosa and bulimia. As noted in the introduction, eating disorders are complex illnesses that are beyond the scope of this book. If you are interested in learning more about these serious, end-stage body-image problems, see appendix D for a list of recommended books on the subject.

BUT . . . DON'T WE NEED TO BEWARE OF FATNESS?

This important question is best answered by a different one: Given the fear of fatness and push for a slim physique that has become a frenzy in the past forty years—with dieting for weight loss now a normal eating style and exercise to burn calories and create "buns of steel" now the rage—have we achieved our goal? Has our fat phobia kept us thin? The statistics to the contrary are mind boggling. Even when adjusted for changing standards, the number of Americans considered overweight has risen from somewhere around 14 percent in the 1960s to over 50 percent today. Obviously something is wrong with our approach. Children grow up today in a culture that holds slimness, especially in women, to be an essential criteria for desirability (ensuring body-image problems), while on the other hand, we grow fatter by the decade (ensuring health-related concerns).

Most of the general public today still embraces dieting, even for teens and children, as a method of weight control, not aware that both research and overwhelming clinical evidence have demonstrated it is counterproductive. Even many physicians have remained uninformed or, in some cases, have discounted the evidence against dieting for weight control. For example, a major study involving nearly 15,000 boys and girls, ages nine through fourteen, reported in the October 2003 *Pediatrics* that dieting for weight loss, even with moderate food restriction, is not only ineffective, but *frequently results in weight gain*. Dieters were significantly more likely than nondieters to report excessive or binge eating following or between diets. During three years of follow-up, dieters in the study gained more weight than nondieters. The more often dieting occurred, the more weight was gained. Despite this scientific cautionary tale, efforts to control weight by cutting calories, or strictly limiting an entire food group, seem more a way of life than ever before. The number of diet books purchased in 2003 far surpassed any prior year in history, and as 2004 rolled in we witnessed a virtual explosion of retailers and restaurants hoping to cash in on the latest low-carb weight-loss mania.

Is this the confusing legacy we want to leave our kids? I don't want my children to suffer the effects of an unhealthy body image *or* an unhealthy body weight. I do not believe in the inevitability of girls' growing up to feel bad about how they look and learning to diet as a rite of passage. You don't either, and that's why you are reading this book. Have you heard the alarm yet? The question is not *whether* to act to prevent body-image and eating concerns, it is how to proceed.

NORMAL DEVELOPMENTAL SEQUENCE FOR ADOLESCENT GIRLS IN AMERICA

After a breathtaking escalation of this problem over recent decades, social scientists have identified a developmental progression that is so common in our daughters, it reliably explains most body-image concerns and body-image-related eating problems. To the degree that our culture is now pressuring males to take on similar beliefs and values about appearance, this explanation may soon apply to boys as well. The good news is that understanding this sequence gives us information about how to prevent it, if we can interrupt it early enough.

The sequence begins with acceptance of the belief that (1) female desirability is determined first and foremost by physical attractiveness and (2) a necessary criterion of physical attractiveness in females is a thin body. This progresses to (3) dissatisfaction with her body: she feels fat or is afraid of becoming fat. In response, she engages in (4) dietary restraint in an effort to lose weight or to maintain an already low weight. This leads to (5) the predictable counterproductive results of dieting: preoccupation with food, increased or ravenous hunger, compulsive or binge eating, weight gain, obsession with weight, and fear of food. In the end she experiences (6) increased distrust of and dissatisfaction with her body. She feels fat (or fatter) and is even more afraid of becoming fat(ter) if she doesn't diet. The cycle then returns to step 1 and begins again with increasing intensity.

From a statistical perspective American girls who do *not* follow the corrosive sequence described are currently *abnormal.* Your daughters may be considered odd if they do *not* feel fat and engage in unhealthy eating as a result of this dissatisfaction. They may be viewed with suspicion (by adults and peers) and possibly even accused of thinking they're better than the rest. You may grasp this paradox more easily if you consider the following:

• It is natural and healthy for girls to add up to 20 percent of their body weight in fat at the time of puberty. (Did you know this? Do you wish you had known this when you were going through puberty?)

- As children enter puberty, it is natural and healthy for them to begin to separate from and identify less with parents, and more with friends. Belonging very often means fitting in with the culture's norms, even at the expense of self.

- A prevalent belief in the wider culture is that female desirability is determined first and foremost by physical attractiveness and that a necessary criterion of physical attractiveness in females is a thin body.

- Therefore, at the same time as a girl's biological nature begins to unfold, as her body begins to naturally round out, her body begins to conflict with the values demanded by her culture and peers—just as the views of that group are becoming critically important to her.

Little wonder pubescent girls join their peers in hating their bodies. Those who don't are outsiders. But this clash of biology with sociology is a recipe for disaster. When we try to help our children to feel comfortable in their bodies, it is critical to remember the pressure children are under to conform. To maintain their health, we are asking them to be different—countercultural even—no small step for any of us, let alone a young adolescent.

This fact brings us full circle to the need to begin prevention earlier than we ever thought necessary and to systematically teach children to maintain body integrity as a matter of course. The changes in appearance that occur with puberty naturally draw children's attention to their bodies. In today's culture, this has signaled a critical shift toward unhealthy body-image attitudes for most girls and some boys. This means that prevention efforts that are first introduced when kids are in middle school are too late. Prevention should begin *before* problems occur.

BUT . . . DON'T FAT CHILDREN
NEED A DIFFERENT APPROACH?

This question reflects a sobering reality that threatens the health and well-being of millions of kids. Children whose bodies are both over the weight that is natural for them and who lack physical fitness are at increased risk for type 2 diabetes and other health problems. In addition, it may be impossible or difficult for them to participate fully in certain physical activities with their peers. If your primary concern is an overweight or obese child, you are still reading the right book. Don't skip to lessons 7 and 8 without first carefully reading all the preceding chapters. Only by understanding the big picture can you be sure to avoid many of the well-intentioned, but tragic mistakes that are often made in the name of weight control. Your wish to help a fat child may lead you to prescribe a weight-loss plan without first taking into full account factors that are likely to defeat your goal.

It is essential to first learn about the limits of our influence over body size and shape, and the limits of our ability to restrain hunger through dieting. We are all bombarded daily with messages (both commercial advertisements and well-meaning health promotions) that state in no uncertain terms that anyone with enough willpower and determination can—and should—lose weight and keep it off. We hear that with weight training and exercise, anyone can sculpt their body into the desired shape.

If you do not first understand the missing qualifiers in these messages—the unwritten fine print—you will inadvertently accept several self-perpetuating myths that may seem to be a solution but that inevitably make things worse.

When you become familiar with what is and what is not within our control about body weight, size, shape, fatness/thinness, hunger, appetite, and activity level, you will have the tools to help any child of any weight succeed at finding her best weight. Then you will be prepared to focus your energy on behaviors that promote health, satisfaction, self-esteem, and well-being.

RESPONDING TO THE ALARM: EFFECTIVE PREVENTION

In chapter 2 I discuss six prevalent cultural myths that encourage body-image and eating problems in American culture. Before we consider these and how to prevent their negative affects, it helps to know what works and what doesn't work when it comes to effective prevention.

No one wants a child to suffer needlessly. We want to protect our kids from harmful influences. We warn them of potential danger. But warning kids about things that could go wrong is not very effective when it comes to prevention. Here's an example: When my kids were starting to drive, my instincts were to say things like, "Don't crash!" I wanted to take them to look at crashed cars and to visit victims in rehabilitation centers. Warnings like these might have driven home the risks of driving. They certainly would relay the intensity of my anxiety! But I knew that wouldn't be helpful, and I bit my tongue. What they really needed were tools for safe driving. I didn't wait until they were calling on a cell phone, headed too fast into a curve on a snowy night to give them these tools. To the contrary, we endlessly reviewed all the things to do instead of risky behavior before they ever left the driveway.

It is the same with prevention of body-image concerns.

Rather than descriptions of emaciated anorexic patients or warnings about unhealthy obesity, we have to prepare our children ahead of time with the tools they need to *maintain body esteem*—especially in the face of bad conditions. We can't wait until kids are rounding the curve into puberty, comparing their bodies and appearance to a cultural "ideal" that virtually ensures they will feel bad about themselves— and then tell them not to do this. We can't wait until they are skipping lunch (and nutrients) trying to achieve this unrealistic slender standard, only to comfort themselves with chocolate and TV when they are disappointed with the results. It is very hard to change negative body image and eating habits once they have begun. We need to stop problems before they start by teaching our kids what to do instead. This is effective prevention.

If you have a child who is already struggling with body image or unhealthy eating habits, do not despair that you are too late. It is never too late to help kids find a better course. It's only that this will take some deprogramming of negative beliefs and behaviors before positive lessons can replace them. The sooner you begin, the easier it will be for your child.

CHAPTER 2

CULTURAL MYTHS AND
THE LOSS OF BODY ESTEEM

C hildren are born with confidence in their bodies. They trust their hunger and their appetites, and rightly so. How does this go wrong?

What forces undermine body esteem, create negative body image, and promote unhealthy eating? Most important, how can we prevent our kids from succumbing to these pressures? The more we learn about what places our kids at risk, the better prepared we will be to help them navigate their preteen and teen years with their body integrity intact.

A CULTURE IS FORMED BY THE
STORIES ITS CHILDREN ARE TOLD

Children hear many stories as they grow up. Ideally, these contain messages that reinforce what it takes to have a happy, healthy life. But unless your kids are extremely isolated, they live in an environment that will also expose them to tales that are not so wholesome. Among these is a set of six cultural myths that actively promote body-image, eating, and weight problems.

In today's media-driven culture, messages routinely instruct us and our children about what we supposedly have to have to be desirable, loveable, and therefore, happy, and how to get the necessary goods to achieve this. One subset of these messages provides lessons specifically about the *look* that is required for this, the *body* that is needed to achieve that look, and *what to do* to get that body. The fact that these directives are at odds with our basic biological nature and deeply conflict with what is needed for physical and emotional well-being is rarely discussed among grown-ups, let alone taught to children. Likewise, it is almost never explained to children that nearly all these messages exist to make money for someone.

Messages about looks are delivered to your children every day without discrimination. None include a label that says, "Warning: Messages regarding the look to have and how to get it are myths that may be hazardous to your physical health and quality of life." Instead, these storylines flow freely, without qualifiers or disclaimers. Neither you nor your children can escape them.

You may think that these messages come only from television, radio, magazines, and movies, and that you can protect your child by controlling your environment. I'm sorry to say this is not possible. Even if you carefully screen what comes into your home, these messages slide by on the sides of buses, beam down from billboards, pop up on computer screens, stare out from bigger-than-life photos displayed in store windows, and display themselves on the covers of magazines at your doctor's office and corner store. Glossy junk-mail messages creep into your mailbox, and flyers are stuck into your front door. The sheer quantity and prevalence of these messages is astonishing.

Experts who study the causes of eating disorders have determined that the accumulation of this set of messages has resulted in a whole new way of thinking about body appearance called the "thinness schema." The thinness schema means that most Americans agree with and identify with the following statements: Beauty is the primary project of a woman's life. A successful woman can and should transform and control herself through fashion, dieting, and rigorous exercise to conform to the desired lean look.

In my talks around the country, I find most people are offended by such superficial statements, at least in theory. But in practice, many of us have to admit we have become carriers of this ideal. Children learn the value of the right body and how to get it not only from the media but when they hear adults greet each other with, "You look great! Have you lost weight?" or, "She's so pretty—too bad about her size." They learn unintentional lessons as they watch us mount scales each morning and count calories each night, or as they see weight-conscious teachers drink diet sodas while skipping lunch. They learn to personalize these messages at the first blush of puberty when well-meaning relatives warn, "Better watch out, you're getting a little pudgy," when teenage siblings complain, "My thighs are gross!" or when they learn that "fat pig" is the worst insult to be hurled on the playground. Even in doctors' offices, destructive messages are too often dispensed through charts that tell children they are over- or underweight, with no regard to other factors that may influence this number.

This chapter explains six prevalent cultural myths that promote the thinness schema and the unhealthy eating habits that accompany it. These myths are tall tales that wrap themselves around and through our lives. Originating only in the last four decades, they have now become so much a part of everyday American life that we hardly notice them, much less question their validity. But they are not benign fairy tales. Rather, they form the basis for much of the weight-obsessed, dieting-and-overeating, all-or-nothing, fat-phobic-but-growing-fatter-by-the-year phenomenon in our society. With the beliefs they teach so woven into the fabric of our lives, we should not be surprised when our smart, eager kids embrace these myths. As you become conscious of these damaging myths in the coming pages, you will also learn the antidotes kids need to resist unhealthy pressures and maintain body esteem via the lessons in part 2.

Myth: "Image is everything. It's not who you are, it's how you look that matters."

Most of us have taught our kids that beauty is only skin deep. We warn them not to judge a book by its cover. So how did the role of external appearance get so out of balance? It turns out there is another adage we have forgotten: One picture is worth a thousand words.

Pictures have been part of the human scene since the Stone Age. But in the early 1950s, a revolutionary age of pictures was ushered in by high-tech cameras, mass production, and mass media. Almost overnight, with programming funded by advertisers, television became affordable for the ordinary person. This period of postwar prosperity saw a huge increase in the publication of glossy magazines and mail-order catalogues. Fashion, beauty, food, home decor, and other themes were aimed particularly at women, most of whom were homemakers with unprecedented levels of disposable income.

To compete with television, the movie industry expanded, in turn fueling waves of star-studded magazines filled with glamorous shots of actors and actresses. Billboards filled with giant pictures began to replace small road signs along our highways. Between 1950 and 1960, visual-imagery rivals ferociously competed for advertiser and viewer attention with ever flashier, bigger, brighter, and more eye-catching appeal. The psychology of how to sell a product became a multibillion dollar industry. The power of a beautiful face and body to convince buyers they needed whatever was being sold created a frenzy of product competition.

I remember the 1950s calendars that Pontiac Motor Company distributed to my father for his automobile dealership—always with pretty women sitting on the hoods of shiny new cars, skirts blowing flirtatiously in a phantom wind. Before the 1960s, this kind of exposure to pictures of movie stars and models in everyday life was still the exception, not the rule. These special-looking people were exactly that: special. As a result, the visual standard against which people routinely compared their own and each other's looks was not unusual or glamorous beauty, but rather other ordinary people.

In today's world, with literally hundreds of glamorous models per day in our line of vision, it is hard to maintain our "ordinary" eye. This is even truer as the finished images that appear in mass media are not ordinary photos. Besides the sheer quantity of handsome men and beautiful women, the quality of their presentation has undergone a dramatic change as well. Today's commercial advertisers choose ever slimmer, perfectly proportioned, photogenic models with exquisitely symmetrical features. These human specimens are then carefully "made over" by use of cosmetics, hair products, cinchers, pads, and boosters. Their photos are artfully crafted with special lighting, flattering camera angles, and other tricks of the trade. Images are enhanced and "perfected" through computerized alterations to eliminate the slightest flaws, intensify or soften the color of eyes, lips, cheeks, and skin, smooth all bumps, wrinkles, blemishes, or freckles, and eliminate inches from a waist or thigh. The end result is an extraordinary virtual reality—an "ideally" seductive human construction that has resulted in a whole new standard of "perfect" external beauty—more a work of art and imagination than a photo of a person.

Yet isn't appreciation of art and beauty part of what makes us human? In fact, people are attracted not only to beauty but to an agreed-upon standard of beauty. While cultural trends influence preferences, there are certain characteristics that nearly all humans find attractive. Studies show that infants, for example, look and smile more at faces that are symmetrical, with features of certain mathematical proportions. So our interest in external physical beauty is built in, and our preference for one look over another is to some degree innate as well.

People have cared about appearance since the beginning of civilization, but never in the self-defeating manner that has gradually consumed us since the onset of mass photo media. The cumulative effect of hundreds upon thousands of these beautiful images en masse capitalizes on this human vulnerability and, in only a few decades, has in many ways changed what children and adults believe is normal and important in life. It is the quality and quantity of these images that has caused our standards to change and our children to embrace two very powerful but dangerous beliefs.

The first belief is that looks are very important. Why else would so many images of similarly "beautiful" people—about whom we know nothing else—surround us at every turn? The second belief is that there is one "right" way to look. Don't the advertisements tell us exactly this?

"Get the right look for back to school, the beach, a night on the town, the office, etc., this year."

"Get the right face,... right hair,... right nails,... the right feet, skin, lips."

"Get a firm tummy, buns of steel, bigger/smaller breasts, the thin thighs you always wanted."

The bottom-line message: Get the look you have to have in order to get whatever else you may want in life. Of course this perspective begs the question: What do you have if you don't have the "right" look?

It's hard to think of another arena in which the line between having what it takes and not having what it takes is so narrow as in the area of looks. We don't talk about the "right" intellect, or athletic, artistic, musical, or mechanical ability. Few of us feel we are complete failures if we have average talent, or are middle income, or normal intelligence. But without the "right" look, we can feel doomed. When your son reaches his teen years, the thin line between the "right" look and the "wrong" one may determine whether he raises his hand in class or hopes to be invisible. It may influence whether or not your daughter will try out for the play, swim club, or basketball team. With the line between the "right" and "wrong" appearance so narrow, virtually everyone, regardless of size or shape, feels deficient at some time.

It is this drain of self-confidence that we hope to help our children avoid.

As a psychotherapist I have worked with several fashion models. Most people have no idea that these attractive women and men often feel inadequate and anxious in real life in comparison to their own enhanced photos. As noted lecturer Jean Kilbourne says of models in advertising, "No one looks like this, not even her!" And yet everything about the model's media image says, "If you buy this product, you can look like me." Some models engage in unhealthy lifestyle habits and develop eating disorders in an effort to achieve or maintain an unnatural body size. Even extremely thin models have told me they were advised to lose weight to be hired.

I have found that girls in seventh and eighth grade often deny that today's mass-media images have any effect on them. They are surprised to hear of a study that tested the impact of advertisements presenting "ideally beautiful" fashion models. Researchers began by administering a self-esteem test to groups of college women. The women then looked at fashion magazines for twenty minutes. When self-esteem was measured again immediately after this viewing, there was a significant drop in these women's scores.

TROUBLE IN PARADISE

Natives of the island country of Fiji have long appreciated more voluptuous women over those who were slender. Three years after cable television (transmitted primarily from the United States) was introduced there in 1995, dieting to lose weight became common among Fijian women. Previously unheard of, 62 percent of teenage Fijian girls reported having dieted and 74 percent said they felt "too big or too fat."

Advertisers aggressively play upon our insecurities and cultivate our wish to be more than we are, leaving us feeling bad about ourselves. The result? Healthy, hungry, normal adults and children compare themselves to fantasies provoked by images and cannot help but feel deficient in comparison. Fortunately there are ways we can intervene. Three lessons in part 2 help your child resist the notion that image is everything:

- Lesson 1 will help your child understand some of the ways in which many of today's unhealthy body-image attitudes and eating habits developed. Your child will gain historical perspective and awareness that things were not always this way.

- Lesson 2 will help you guide your child to keep looks in balance and to remember appearance is only one part of who they are.

- Lesson 9 will show you how to help your son or daughter become media literate and to resist advertisements that sell a "right" way to look.

Myth: "Fatter people are overweight."

As the emphasis on external image has increased, fads about the desired look have been accepted as mandates. The "right" look is perceived as essential—something we have to have. When it comes to body size and shape, what was once a preference for a slim body has become a *demand* for a slim body. With thinness now considered to be a necessary criteria for desirability, the belief that fatter bodies are "wrong" has evolved. Fatter people (of any degree) are now assumed to be overweight.

Children as young as five believe that fatter people eat too much and that they eat more than other people. As a culture, we believe that all people with observable fat are over the weight that they should be and that they most certainly could do something about it if they tried.

Imagine two high school girls, both slender, but one four-foot-eleven and the other six feet tall. Whether these girls appreciate or disdain the extremes of their height, it would be unheard of for anyone to say to them, "You really should do something about your height." This is because we rarely argue with bones. We may *prefer* a different height, longer fingers, smaller feet, but most of us spend little time trying to actually change these structural parts of ourselves. I remember in fourth grade longing for a turned-up nose like that of my best friend. For about a week I sat at my school desk, pinky finger crooked over the bridge of my nose, pushing down, hoping to reshape it. Then . . . I gave up! It didn't take long to realize, like it or not, that I had little choice but to live with the nose I had been given. In the same way, most tall and short girls make peace with their height.

Now imagine another girl, five-foot-six and 175 pounds. The average American would describe her as overweight. We would not say so out loud, but most would think, "Well, she *is* pretty fat. She really should go on a diet." Why do we assume the heavy girl should alter her eating and "do something about her weight" in contrast to the two slim girls? Do we know that the tall and short girls have healthy lifestyles? Maybe they have high metabolism rates, but are totally out-of-shape couch potatoes who eat nothing but low-nutrient junk food. Maybe they are slim because they have eating disorders. Do we know that the heavy girl does *not* have wholesome eating habits? Maybe she is a triathlete with the best eating habits and highest fitness level of the three. In truth, our presumptuous judgment that the fatter girl should do something about her weight is based on external appearance alone. All or none of these girls may be healthy and fit.

Taking this a step further, in a routine medical checkup, it's unlikely that these girls would have either their eating habits or level of physical fitness assessed. Yet even in the absence of this information, it would not be surprising if the larger girl were told to begin a weight-loss plan. Such a prescription, based on the assumption that she must be doing something wrong to account for her fatter figure, fails to consider that there are many factors that account for diverse body weight. The truth is that from 50 to 80 percent of the influence for body size and shape is genetic or otherwise driven by internal weight regulatory mechanisms that are outside of our control. This includes not only genetic predisposition for bone structure but also fat-to-lean-tissue composition, the location of fat stores, and metabolic rate.

I am certainly not suggesting we have no influence over weight. We have not become the fattest nation on earth because of a change in our genetic predisposition. This elementary biology lesson, however, does expose popular myths that propose we have a *lot* of control over our weight. The truth is, bodies are hardwired from birth to *defend* a set-point weight range that is "normal" or "right" for us by way of a highly complex internal system. Like the thermostat in your home, this regulatory system directs metabolism, appetite, the kinds of foods we prefer, and other factors in order to maintain or return the body to its natural, stable degree of fatness or thinness at each stage of life. If we all satisfied our hunger with the same, wholesome food and achieved an equal level of physical fitness, our bodies would still be very diverse—short to tall, and lean to fat.

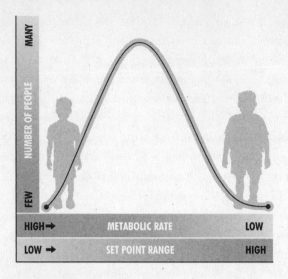

It is true that bodies can be forced to add or drop weight above or below our set-point range. At the same time, research confirms what we see in everyday life. To fatten someone above her defended set point or to slim her below this range requires unhealthy means. Given healthy habits, some people "eat like a horse" and never gain a pound, while others eat sparingly and remain fat. If weight is above or below the set-point range *because of unhealthy eating and lifestyle habits*, then healthy habits (not under- or overeating) will help restore the natural weight range, whether that is fatter or thinner.

All of us will benefit from understanding the myth that assumes fat people inevitably eat too much and exercise too little, and that thin people are fit, healthy eaters. Especially as they are filling out in puberty, it's important for kids to know that diverse body shapes are natural and that it's not possible to know if someone is overweight, underweight, or at their natural weight just by looking at them. In part 2 you will find three lessons with activities that will help you convey this.

- The activities in lesson 3 will help your child understand that genetics are the greatest determinant of body size and shape. Together, you can consider his or her own biological heritage.

- Lesson 4 emphasizes that with proper care, each person's internal weight regulatory system will help him maintain a weight that is natural and healthy for him.

- Lesson 5 will help you prepare your child ahead of time for the many different, but normal ways that bodies will grow and appearances will change during puberty.

Myth: "Fatter people are undesirable or bad."

A few years ago someone sent me a greeting card with a cartoon that has a male and female dinosaur, both dressed for an evening out as they stand facing each other. She also wears a look that would kill as he naively says to her, "That dress kinda makes you look fat." The caption: *"The REAL reason dinosaurs are extinct!"*

Why do most of us, including me, think this cartoon is funny? Would it prompt a laugh in a culture in which fatness is considered to be attractive? Of course not. The humor in this punch line is dependent on our shared understanding that telling someone they look fat is an insult.

Our belief that fatness is preventable and that anyone with a little willpower can be slim is routinely used to justify our prejudices about it. Studies show that people who are fat are thought of as undesirable, lazy, stupid, dirty, and jolly but unhappy. On the other hand, slender, lean people are judged to be virtuous, admirable, energetic, intelligent people who have it all together. Children as young as five believe fatter people are inferior and less deserving of equal rights (equal time on the swing set, or to be first in line for lunch, etc.). Indeed, children commonly use "fat" as a general-purpose putdown, even when the person being slammed is skinny.

There is no aspect of appearance in which the dividing line between acceptable and unacceptable is so narrow as in our judgment of fatness versus thinness. From slim and desirable to fat and gross can be a hairsbreadth. Five pounds can shift us from "looking good" to "ugly pig." Smart, pure, and desirable can become stupid, gross, and unwanted between the Thanksgiving turkey and the New Year's Eve resolution to "never eat again!"

Weight prejudice, or weightism, is no different from racism, sexism, or ageism. With any ism, negative judgments are based on ignorance, assumptions, and generalizations, rather than facts. Labels are assigned based on external characteristics. Even when these have statistical probability (for example, the assumption that a seven-foot-tall athlete is a basketball player), it is still presumptuous. When the judgment is negative, it is destructive. Prejudicial responses deny people their individuality, and sometimes their basic rights. Yet the ignorance upon which weightism is based is so common that we rarely question, let alone challenge it. Jokes that ridicule fat people go unopposed since most people, even many who are fat themselves, assume these put-downs are deserved.

There is more prejudice about body size in the United States than any other single target of prejudice. Our language offers many good illustrations of this. The best example is our use of the word *overweight*. If a person with healthy eating habits and good aerobic fitness is fat, then what weight are they over? Are they over the weight that is right for them? Concern for the potential health risks of fatness often serves as a mask for weightism. Once a person is labeled "overweight" we immediately begin to assume a corrective response is needed. On the other hand, unless an individual is approaching emaciation, our response to a diagnosis of "underweight" (even for those with anorexia) may be closer to envy and admiration than concern.

While medical concerns related to the rising weight of our nation's population are warranted, rampant negative judgments about fatness will not help to improve the health or quality of life of Americans. Scorn and degradation have never been effective change agents. In my clinical practice I have worked with many fat-bodied women, men, and children who will assure you that weightist attitudes will not reduce their girth or the waistline of America.

Adults who have grown up with the word *fat* as an insult will find it difficult (maybe even impossible) to rid themselves of this prejudice. For your children's sake, you may initially need to settle for suppressing your conditioned response to fatness while outwardly presenting a more tolerant and open attitude. On a hopeful note, we have learned from experience in the classroom that when young children are taught that even if they have a *preference* for slimness, this does not justify a judgment about fatness, they are able to embrace a much more accepting stance. Children who hear words descriptive of body sizes that are used nonjudgmentally can and do learn to do the same. Our job is to make sure this is what they hear and to challenge weightism whenever it appears.

All of the lessons in part 2 will help you to use words that describe body size and shape in nonjudgmental ways with your kids. Here are some examples you can use when your children ask specific questions about fatness or weight. Otherwise you can simply look for opportunities to use loaded words (like *fat*) without judgment.

Why is Mr. Riley so fat? Look at that fat lady! Is Grandma fat?
Some people are naturally thinner. Some people are naturally fatter. For example, I'm fatter than Aunt Mary is, but thinner than Aunt Sue. Now, your grandmother is fat in her bottom but thin in her top—just like your great-grandma. We are all thinner than Mr. Riley, but have you noticed Mr. Riley rides his bike everywhere, every day? Plus he eats all those vegetables he grows in his garden. From what I know about Mr. Riley, he's probably very healthy. The important thing is that we all eat well and exercise a lot. This means we can be confident we are the size we were meant to be.

But isn't it wrong to be fat?
It's not right or wrong to be fat. If a person eats well, is strong and fit, and their body is still fat, how can that be wrong? But if a person doesn't eat nutritious food and doesn't get any exercise, then that could be bad for their health, even if they are thin. Eating well and staying fit are the right things to do for your health, regardless of the size you turn out to be.

Am I fat? What if I get fat? I'm so fat!
How much fatness do you think would be natural for you? Kids often get fatter before they get taller when they go through puberty. Girls can add 20 percent of their body weight in fat during puberty. Do you eat nutritious food?

Are you strong and fit? If so, then you can be sure your size is probably just right for you.

Myth: "When it comes to weight, dieting is the cure for the wrong body."

"Where there's a will, there's a way." There is a lot of value in this enthusiastic attitude, which we try to instill in our children. Unfortunately, we don't always remember that there are limits. While hard work and determination will take us a long way, we cannot do, be, or have whatever we put our minds to. Sometimes things outside of our control affect our options.

It is apparent that many people do not accept the limits of their genetic makeup when 75 percent of America's females dislike their bodies. But when it comes to weight, there is another way we deny the limits to our control: our belief that *dieting is the cure for the wrong body*.

The word *diet* can be used to describe any eating plan, including a wholesome diet, rich in nutritious foods. When I use the word *dieting*, however, I mean the following: *Restricted eating according to an external plan that prescribes not only what but how much to eat for the purpose of losing weight*. Compare this to an adapted definition of "normal eating" offered by author and dietitian Ellyn Satter: *Satisfaction of internal hunger cues with a balanced variety of foods that over time fulfill nutritional needs and personal taste preferences*.

For several decades the scientific community has understood that external restriction of food is not an effective weight-loss strategy; the most important research on this topic was completed over fifty years ago! Unfortunately, articles reporting this conclusion to the general public have only trickled out in recent years. By now most people have read something about the inadvisability of dieting, and yet we persist in it. In fact, dieting for weight loss is a statistically normal eating style in America and a booming multibillion-dollar industry. Why do we continue to engage in these self-defeating weight-loss efforts?

One reason is that we are told to diet. When I was interviewing a class of fifth graders recently, I showed them a slide filled with diet headlines such as "Lose Weight Fast!" "Get Our Revolutionary New Weight-Loss Bullet," "Drop Ugly Pounds Now," etc. I asked the children how frequently they saw advertisements like these. Without hesitation they answered, "Every day! All the time!" If you and your children are exposed to the outside world in any way, it is unlikely you will go through a single day without being told to lose weight through dieting.

It's critical that you recognize an aspect of pervasive diet advertisements that is particularly dangerous for children: Diet ads almost never identify their target audience. *"Lose Weight Now!"* applies to *anyone* and, therefore, by default, *everyone*, regardless of age or whether there is even any actual weight to lose. Taken at face value, every one of us, including our children, should *"Drop 2 Sizes by Summer!"* Teachers say they are too often shocked to hear first- and second-grade students say, "I need to go on a diet." Where do kids get this idea? Remember the preponderance of advertisements urging weight loss. How will your children know that these ads are not for them? Stricter guidelines for diet advertisements are imperative. In the meantime, we have our work cut out for us.

A second reason people continue to diet is that diets work—in the short run. If we cut enough calories, regardless of the method, we lose weight. "Lose 30 pounds in 30 days!" is an extremely unhealthy plan, but you will drop pounds if you actually follow it. It's hard to argue with visible success. If we have been feeling fat, joining the program can be very tempting when we see our friends and neighbors dropping pounds. What we forget (or maybe never knew) is that *95 percent of all weight that is lost through any type of dieting is regained in the first year, usually with additional pounds.*

The more extreme the diet and the faster the loss, the faster the regain. But even those who choose healthier and less extreme diets can expect to gradually regain pounds that are lost through calorie restriction. To recap: *Dieting for weight loss is not effective.*

Nonetheless, dieting continues unabated in the United States, perhaps because most people don't understand why diets are counterproductive. When weight is regained by dieters, most people still blame "lack of willpower" rather than understanding the plan is fatally flawed. Hundreds of my clients, representing thousands of pounds lost and regained (usually multiple times), introduced themselves to me with shame. Virtually every one insisted their dieting failure was due to gluttony and lack of willpower, or their "addiction" to food. What they didn't know is that there are predictable, counterproductive results that occur when eating is restricted according to an external plan. In part 2 you will learn what is behind this cause-and-effect equation in a fun exercise you can do with your children:

- Lesson 6 will help you teach your child why dieting for weight loss is not a good idea. Dieters lose weight at first, but eventually almost all regain it—probably with added pounds *and* added hunger in the future.

Myth: "Fatness is a health risk for which weight loss can be prescribed."

Fatness that is the result of too much high-calorie, low-nutrient eating and a too-sedentary lifestyle poses a serious health risk. This kind of fatness decreases the quality of life and life expectancy for an increasing number of people. In fact, at today's rate of growth, America would achieve 100 percent obesity by 2230. The unprecedented fattening of America is a monumental problem, and without learning ways to reverse this trend we cannot promote body esteem in our children.

At the same time, we need to pay attention to new, compelling research that challenges our basic assumptions about the relationship between weight and health. Important studies in the past decade have revealed that fatter people who are fit are at significantly lower risk for weight-related health problems than thinner people who are not fit. One such study included 25,389 people who were followed for over five years. These reports raise a new question: Is it fatness or lack of fitness that poses the health risk? Fortunately, for those of us who just want our families to be healthy, the answer isn't needed. Whether the culprit is fatness or lack of fitness, the practical question is the same: What can be prescribed for improved health as well as overall quality of life?

Weight control and/or weight loss are routinely recommended. But what can we actually *control* about weight over the long haul? Consider this parallel example: If you are male, then you are at a higher risk for certain illnesses than females: early heart disease, prostate cancer, and accidental death, just to name a few. Females are at higher risk for other illnesses: osteoporosis, autoimmune diseases, breast cancer, and migraine headaches, for example. But male or female, when you see your physician, how often does she look you in the eye and say, "You know, with the added risk, you really should do something about your gender"?

Your doctor would not purposefully recommend you change something that is not in your power to change. Instead, he or she automatically accounts for the risk factors that are outside of your control and then prescribes actions you can take that may reduce health risks. Receiving regular cholesterol checks, quitting smoking, eating more calcium-rich foods, or reducing stress might be advised.

When it comes to weight, we seem to forget there are built-in factors that may interfere with a prescription for permanent weight loss. When we remember to consider genetic predisposition, the weight regulatory system, and the ineffectiveness of dieting, what choices remain? Realistically, there are only two options. We can choose what to eat to satisfy hunger, and we can decide on the degree to which we are active or sedentary throughout our lives.

Let's say we decide to go for the best possible outcome and commit to *improve* our less-than-perfect habits. We begin to eat in a very wholesome manner and achieve a high degree of physical fitness through regular physical activity. We would all be much healthier as a result. New research assures us that even modest improvements in nutrition and exercise can significantly reduce health risks. But would we all be slim? Could we all expect to lose weight as a result of these lifestyle improvements? By now you know the answer is no, we could not.

This is so important that it bears repeating. *We can count on improved health, but not everyone can count on a slim or even slimmer appearance (or body mass index) as a result of eating well and choosing an active, even aerobic lifestyle.*

Most people who have gained weight as a result of unhealthy lifestyle choices *would* lose weight with improved habits. But some people will lose little or no weight at all. They will become healthier—maybe a lot healthier. But they may not lose weight. The truth is, other than through extraordinary means (such as surgical or pharmaceutical interventions) we cannot *prescribe* a lasting goal weight because weight can be influenced by choices, but not controlled. Given healthy choices, natural weight will be revealed for each one of us over time and will range from naturally slim to naturally fat.

When an editorial in the *New England Journal of Medicine* recommended that physicians stop prescribing weight loss and instead urge their patients to eat well and become physically fit, it caused an uproar. Former surgeon general Dr. C. Everett Koop reported that this approach would lead to a "don't worry, be flabby" mentality in the American public. While well intentioned, Dr. Koop's response reflects a lack of understanding of the seeds of complacency. If a person does all the right things and still doesn't get the promised reward (in this case, weight loss or a goal weight), it is a prescription for failure. Offering slimness as the "reward" for a healthy lifestyle has backfired, resulting in the complacency we hoped to avoid:

"Why should I eat healthy if it doesn't make me thin?" (fourteen-year-old girl)

"I exercised five days a week for three months and I still didn't lose any weight. What's the use?" (twenty-seven-year-old mother of three)

"When I eat good and get out walking with my neighbor every day, my weight drops to two hundred every time and

stays right there. I feel good! But then I see my doctor. He just looks at me and shakes his head. Then he says, 'You've got to lose more weight.' It's enough to make me cry. I give up." (forty-seven-year-old woman, now 273 pounds)

When people are asked to name their number one motivator for eating healthily and exercising, the most common answer is to "lose weight." Could the discouraged attitudes reflected in the above statements actually contribute to the unhealthy fattening of our nation? In our all-or-nothing, image-is-everything, dieting-for-the-right-body world, disillusionment can be just around the corner for anyone. Add to this the ordinary pressures of everyday life—days full to the brim with school, jobs, activities, family ties, community service, and social schedules—and it can be hard to find the time or energy to reflect, plan, nurture, and nourish our bodies and souls. Instead of looking for satisfaction in a better balance, it is tempting to seek comfort in the quick, easy, generally cheap and readily available solutions offered by one final myth.

Myth: "Eat, drink, and be merry. Healthy choices are just too much work!"

Eating for sheer pleasure and comfort is enjoyable for most of us. "Eat, drink, and be merry," however, too frequently means sacrificing long-term health, physical strength, and well-being for the momentary respite of short-term indulgence. Feeling guilty is not helpful. A sympathetic understanding is more realistic. With the array of cheap, mouthwatering, readily available comfort foods and sedentary-entertainment options, few adults, let alone children, can resist. With the average child viewing more than forty thousand TV advertise-ments urging them to spend their hunger on high-calorie en-tertainment foods and soda, parents face an uphill battle trying to run a wholesome kitchen. Unfortunately, the un-precedented climb in rates of obesity, type 2 diabetes, eating disorders, and other childhood-health problems is testimony to the fact that we are losing the battle. What can we do when we are up against this kind of pressure?

As parents, we teach our children to be competent in many ways. We guide them to budget their time, work hard, and delay gratification in order to be good students, be strong ath-letes, or finish a work of art. We help them know the value of saving for a bike, sharing with others, and caring for the family pet. All of these take not only good intentions but planning ahead, self-discipline, and follow-through. With all the competencies we teach our children, we may not have re-alized the importance of or known how to teach them to be competent in the care and feeding of their bodies. Given to-day's pressures, this is essential.

Helping our kids maintain body esteem includes teaching them realistic prescriptions for health and how to compe-tently carry these out. In part 2 you will find three lessons to help with this task.

- In Lesson 7 you will find help to encourage your kids to invest their hunger in wholesome foods that provide the balance of nutrients they need.
- Lesson 8 will show your kids that a physically active lifestyle is an essential ingredient for health.
- When your child eats well and is physically fit, you will all discover the size and weight that nature intended. Lesson 10 will help you guide her in choosing positive, realistic role models that will help her accept and feel good about this.

PART TWO

TEN ESSENTIAL LESSONS

✳

I t's not enough to warn children to "just say no" to unwholesome or risky attitudes and behaviors. They need a
guide that helps them to know what to do instead of succumbing to negative pressures. They need a new model for
healthy body image, eating, and lifelong fitness. The Ten Essential Lessons that follow provide a positive approach, giving
you the necessary background information, tips for conversations with your child, stories that reinforce body esteem, and
activities to develop a foundation for healthy body image, eating, and weight.

It is likely that many readers of this book face their own internal body-image demons. You may be a chronic dieter or an
obsessive exerciser. Or, at the opposite extreme, you may have
a hard time finding sufficient energy or interest for healthy
eating and physical fitness. If you struggle with any of the
Ten Essential Lessons, you are in good company. But if you
can embrace these lessons for yourself, do it! If you cannot,
then take heart in teaching and reinforcing what your child
needs, so she or he will not have to carry the same burden.

Parents often ask me whether they should be honest about their own current body-image struggles. This can be a difficult question, especially for moms who are often both primary providers of food for the family and the primary victims of body-image problems. We cannot escape the fact that our kids will learn more from what they see us *do* than from what we *say*. So, for example, children of smokers are more likely to smoke, regardless of the number of times they hear their parents say, "I'm hooked, but you don't have to be." When it comes to body image and a healthy lifestyle, if your kids hear you scorning your body, observe that you are afraid to sit down and eat normally, or notice that you are a compulsive exerciser, this *will* have an effect on them. Likewise, if you rarely eat a vegetable and spend most of your free time on the couch, this will have an impact as well.

As a parent, I know how hard it can be to try to help kids become all they can be in spite of our limitations. My hope is that you can use the Ten Essential Lessons to exorcise your own body-image demons, for your own sake and for that of your children. In the meantime, the more you can keep your painful body-image struggles and diets under wraps, the better.

In a way, this book is really aimed at you, the parent. Since you are your child's first and most profound teacher, the more you absorb and integrate the lessons, the better able you will be to pass on their messages in a natural way. There's no need to set up a quasiclassroom atmosphere to discuss the material. Instead, introduce the concepts so that they flow from whatever is already happening in your family life. For example, after a family reunion, you might suggest the fun follow-up activity from lesson 3: drawing a family tree to discover all the diverse physical characteristics displayed in a single extended family. Or instead of the usual bedtime story, you could read the parable from lesson 1, setting the stage for some impromptu but relevant conversation.

Use "found time" with your child to talk about body-image lessons. You have probably already discovered that driving time together is a great opportunity to casually bring up topics you want to discuss. So is time spent in doctors' and dentists' waiting rooms, at the dinner table, and during walks to the park. When you are primed to take notice, you will find the world around you offers a multitude of opportunities to talk about this subject—advertisements on billboards, radio or TV commercials, slogans on buses, posters at the bus stop, flyers delivered to your mailbox, magazine covers at the grocery store, friends and neighbors revealing their body-image attitudes or announcing their latest diet. You will have many chances to say, "That reminds me . . . ," "What do you think about . . . ?" "Did you know . . . ?" or "I have something I want to show you."

In general, taking your cue from your child will yield the most positive results. Timing does matter, as does your child's mood of the moment. Some topics are too important to let slide, however, and if the time never seems right, you may need to put the topic on the table.

EIGHT TIPS FOR
TEACHING THE LESSONS

1. Read all of the Ten Essential Lessons ahead of time.

This book presents a perspective that is different from the way most Americans have come to think about body size and shape, the role of mass media, and, to some degree, the purpose of eating and exercise. I strongly recommend that you read *all* of the lessons and become familiar with the overall content before you begin to introduce the lessons to your children. If you know where you are going from the start, when you get sidetracked in conversations with your kids (which you surely will), you can better decide what to do next. You may want to say, "That's a good topic for another day," choose to rearrange the order in which you discuss the lessons, or be better prepared to respond to a question that is answered by what you have already read from a later lesson.

2. Teach all of the lessons.

All of the Ten Essential Lessons are needed to understand how to maintain body esteem in today's culture. Many well-intentioned groups have focused on one aspect of the lessons at the expense of another and, in doing so, have actually *contributed* to many of the problems we have today with body image, eating, and weight. Until recently, those concerned with the prevention of eating disorders, overweight and obesity, and acceptance of size diversity have sometimes been at odds with each other. "Solutions" for one problem have too often reinforced other problems. Things are looking brighter since, as I write this, the U.S. Senate has decided to rework a new bill that originally targeted obesity as an isolated health priority into one that mentions eating disorders every time that obesity is mentioned. This far-more-balanced message and realistic approach was highlighted by Senator Clinton in her floor speech:

> *While it is so important to fight the obesity epidemic, we should not inadvertently send the wrong message by telling our children and adults simply to eat less and ex-*

ercise. Unfortunately, many adolescents misinterpret this as a message that they should eat to achieve the body of a runway model. Anorexia and bulimia are increasingly common among our nation's youth.

On page 233 in appendix B is the Model for Healthy Body Image that depicts how these ten lessons fit together, reflecting what can and cannot be controlled about body size and shape. Printable versions are available at www.bodyimagehealth.org.

3. Do the activities.

Most people learn better by doing. While tips for conversations with your child are a part of each lesson, the activities are where the real learning happens. Do them yourself, and you will see the difference. All of the activity worksheets may be photocopied, or you may obtain printable versions from www.bodyimagehealth.com.

4. Look for opportunities to reinforce these lessons in everyday life.

Be prepared to point out and repeat concepts throughout the growing-up years.

5. Share this book with others.

I developed my *Healthy Body Image* curriculum with some ulterior motivation. I wanted my daughter to hear healthy messages from others besides me, in a context that included her peers, and to have these messages reinforced by her friends and their families. If you give or recommend this book to the parents of your child's friends, your school, your pediatrician, the director of your child's ballet school, your child's gymnastics or wrestling coach, or others who are instrumental in your child's life, you will be helping everyone, including your child. You might want to organize a small group of parents to read this book together for support and discussion.

6. Take an active role in protecting your child from adverse messages.

You cannot prevent your child from exposure to unhealthy, unrealistic messages, which is why these lessons aim to develop your child's ability to resist them. But you will send a positive message if you limit exposure to these messages by not bringing fashion magazines into your home (or by not allowing your child to subscribe to them), by screening other media exposure, and by speaking up about the soda and candy vending machines in your child's school—to name a few examples.

7. Model a healthy lifestyle.

Like it or not, we are primary role models for what it means to be a grown-up. If necessary, challenge yourself to demonstrate the same kind of positive, healthy balance in your life that you want for your kids.

8. Be an activist.

There is a list of organizations in the back of this book if you'd like to become more involved. For example, Dads and Daughters is routinely successful at taking on advertisers that portray girls and women in a demeaning light or that encourage disordered eating. Congress acted in response to conversations with advocates from the Eating Disorders Coalition for Research, Policy & Action to rewrite the above-mentioned Senate bill that includes both obesity and eating disorders as priorities. There are even organizations that sponsor activism activities for your child, such as Turn Beauty Inside Out, sponsored annually by *New Moon Magazine for Girls.*

Lesson 1:
Maintain Perspective
IT DOESN'T HAVE TO BE THIS WAY

Body dissatisfaction is so common today, it's easy to forget that only a few decades ago this was not the norm. Compared to the 75 percent of American women who currently struggle with feeling fat, only 30 to 35 percent fell into this group in the 1960s. Hardly any statistics are available prior to that time, presumably because there was little pressing need to gather them. Almost overnight, it has become "normal" for girls to be anxious about their size and worried that eating will make them fat. Our children have no way of knowing it does not have to be this way—unless we tell them.

Our culture is not the only one in which destructive attitudes and behaviors have become the custom. Think about the similarities between today's body-image attitudes and the following examples:

- Until 1911, bound feet were considered to be essential for females in China. The painful binding, maintained from age four until feet were fully grown, aimed to create three-inch "lotus feet," rendering a girl's feet practically useless and confining women to home. At first practiced by only the very rich, the custom spread over the years to even poor farming families. Unbound girls were considered unsuitable for marriage.

- Brass spiral rings of increasing length are still placed on girls' necks in the Pa Dong hill tribe in northern Thailand to prevent them from marrying outside the tribe. Rings force down the girls' ribs as they grow, making their necks appear very long. The "longneck women," who wear the

rings into old age, defend this custom, saying it is "tradition."

- During the nineteenth century corsets were laced so
tightly, wearers could scarcely breathe. The use of the
corset was driven by the social expectation that women
have a fashionable figure, and girls as young as two to four
years of age were trained in their wearing. While not all
women were expected to be slim, laces were drawn tight
enough to create an hourglass shape, supposedly an indica-
tion that the wearer took her appearance seriously.

Whether you consider these practices to be more or less extreme than those resulting from today's body-image norms,
it's useful to think about how such obviously destructive
ideals can be embraced by an entire culture. When your
child learns that today's unrealistic body image and eating
attitudes have developed only re-
cently and understands how these
cause unhappiness, she will be
motivated to learn there is a
healthier alternative.

Because mass media is so persuasive in appealing to our human needs, it is essential that children learn to think critically about the messages that are promoted. Healthy awareness will help us resist idealizing and comparing ourselves to unrealistic standards.

The following story of the Namuh is an engaging parable that
will gently introduce your child to
some of the ways this has happened in our culture. This tale
may seem obvious to adults, but
kids relate closely to the fictitious
society and absorb the important
lessons the Namuh learn. The ex-
perience of the Namuh reveals how a group of well-
intentioned but misguided people can unwittingly develop

values and behaviors that are destructive to them. The Namuh demonstrate many of the ways that negative body-image attitudes and eating behaviors develop. Happily, the story also reveals that a far better way is possible. All of the key concepts that are covered in lessons 2 through 10 are introduced through the Namuh's experience, setting the stage for future discussions about cultural pressures that promote negative body esteem.

It would probably dawn on you that *Namuh* is *human* spelled backward. You will want to keep this to yourself, either until your child discovers it for herself or until you discuss the story at the end. At that time, you can ask your child if she can figure out why the author called these people the Namuh. Recognizing the origin of this name (with your help, if necessary) will increase your child's identification with the Namuh—as well as her desire to avoid the unhappiness they suffered. She will realize the powerful lesson: negative body esteem is not inevitable for her or for anyone who maintains perspective in the face of unhealthy body-image norms.

How the Namuh Learned to
Be Content with Who They Were

Once upon a time in a world not really so far away, lived the Namuh, who happened to be quite a lot like us. The Namuh had their share of life's ups and downs, with good days and bad, happy times and sad. But they had learned to take the good with the bad and understood what they could and could not control. They were content.

One day in the world of the Namuh a photographer was feeling a bit down. He wished to become a very successful photographer. He hoped to sell many portraits, so he could make a lot of money and afford to live in a big house. He was a good man, and good at his business too. Even so, he felt his business was not growing as much as he would like. He needed a new idea to attract people to his photo studio.

Now the Namuh took great pride in their family heritage, and family portraits from many generations before hung on their walls. The photographer thought and thought, until he decided to show off some of his best family portraits in the front window of his store. He hoped the Namuh passing by would like them so much that they would want a portrait of their own family. He also decided to try something that had not been done before. He paid the newspaper, which until then had no pictures, to print some of his best photos. This way all the readers of the newspaper would see his good work and be inspired to have their portrait taken. He carried out his plan, and sure enough, his business doubled in no time!

Customers came from far and wide. Many said it was not the portraits of the grown-up Namuh that had caught their eye in his advertisements. No, it was the portraits of cute, smiling children they oohed and aahed about. The photographer continued to advertise his photos, but more and more he used photos of beautiful young children—for that is what brought in the business.

Time went by, and the photographer was doing very well. Nevertheless, he wanted to do even better. He was only taking pictures of children. He needed to expand his business. He thought, "Young and cute are what Namuh like to look at. Think about it: baby monkeys, kittens, puppies, human babies—big eyes in a little face, sweet little mouths, turned-up noses, soft smooth skin. Now doesn't it just make you smile to imagine it? And when Namuh see what they like, they want to own something like it for themselves. That's it!

Young and fresh and delicate and smooth and perfect, without any lumps or bumps or wrinkles!"

When the photographer realized this, smart man that he was, he had a new idea. "What if I took photos of grown-ups to advertise my business, but chose only those rare grown-ups who still have the youngest-looking faces, with smooth skin, delicate features, and turned-up noses? In my studio, I can make them look perfect with special lights and cosmetics. And they'll have very slim, childlike bodies—tall, but not really rounded, the way most Namuh women are, so they'll look even slimmer! Then other adults will want me to take their pictures too, and my business will double!"

But then he thought, "Would people like grown-up Namuh men to appear cute, like little boys? Hmmm." Namuh usually liked their men to be big and strong so they could work on the farms. He decided to concentrate only on photos of youthful and cute grown-up female Namuh. He was sure this would succeed.

The photographer paid the newspaper to print his advertisements and settled back to see if his idea would work. Sure enough, people flocked to his business. They oohed and aahed about his beautiful photos of the grown-up Namuh females. They wanted their own portraits to look that way.

The photographer was doing very, very well. He bought a big, big house and a different car for every day of the week. He was happy.

Now, one day a neighbor, who had a toothpaste factory, met him on the street. "How do you do it?" he asked—for he wished he could do as well with his toothpaste sales. Since the photographer was a good man, he decided to share his idea with the toothpaste maker. "Cute," he said. "You've got to make your toothpaste cute! That's what I did!"

The toothpaste maker had his doubts, but he didn't think the photographer would steer him the wrong way. So he went back to his factory and set to work. Soon he had the photographer take pictures of his toothpaste tube all dressed up, with little legs and arms sticking out and a big toothy smiling face on the front! Oh, it was cute! He advertised his toothpaste in all the newspapers and magazines, and on the TV too. Sure enough, his sales increased. But not as much as he had hoped.

Time went by. One day the toothpaste maker was having lunch with some business friends: a car maker, a clothing salesperson, a lawn-furniture designer, and an orange-juice salesperson. Who should walk into the restaurant but the photographer! "Join our table," he said to the photographer, hoping to ask for more advice. "I've had success with my cute packaging, but not as much good fortune as you. What do you think I should do?"

The photographer was happy to help if he could. So he thought and he thought. Finally he said, "Maybe it's not cute packaging or cute songs so much as cute, young children or beautiful young-looking women that attract people to buy. Maybe you need to have photos of cute children or young, perfectly beautiful smiling women holding your toothpaste in your advertisement. Then people will feel if they buy your toothpaste, their smiles will look forever young and fresh, like the images of the models in the pictures!"

All the businesspeople showed up at his studio the very next day. And so, the photographer took pictures of toothpaste, orange juice, cars, tennis rackets, and lawn furniture, all arranged with lovely, slim young women who had that special childlike appeal, which he made even more appealing and perfect with his special effects. But it was what happened next that the photographer never, ever could have imagined.

By now the advertisements with unusual models were everywhere: on TV, in newspapers, in magazines, on billboards, on the product labels themselves. The lovely ladies in all the ads all seemed to be saying the same thing: "Look at me! If you buy this product, you'll be as appealing and special as I am!"

It wasn't long before all the Namuh women began to notice that all the models looked one certain way. They were a lot like young fluffy kittens or playful, happy puppies or rosy-cheeked, soft-skinned children—people just couldn't get enough of looking at them. Movie and TV-show makers had caught on too, so now almost all the actresses were chosen for that same young and perfect look. Whenever people looked at pictures of them they oohed and aahed, and felt happy.

At first the female Namuh enjoyed the images of the rare and beautiful Namuh women as much as anyone. Oh, some of them thought it would be fun to look like the models in the ads and on the TV, but they knew most women didn't really look like that.

But as years went by and the ads with the rare Namuh models were everywhere, the feelings of the young Namuh women began to change. Seeing those pictures of beautiful women smiling at them almost from the day they were born . . . well, the Namuh women began to think that maybe that was the way they were supposed to look!

After a while, it came to be that the young Namuh girls no longer remembered that there was a time when there were many different ways to look and that all Namuh had been happy to be who they were. Now most Namuh girls grew up to believe they should compare their looks to the models and look forever young, slim, and perfect.

Of course, almost none of them could look as perfect as

the models. So naturally they could not help feeling bad about themselves in comparison. But when the Namuh females compared themselves to how completely slim and trim the models were, they saw an opportunity. You can't change your skin, your face, or your height—but if you eat less, you can lose weight. Isn't that right?

It wasn't long before more and more of the Namuh women were on strict diets to be thinner. In fact, everyone was so hopeful that diets would give them a slim body like the beautiful models, just about every female was dieting. Since almost no one was as naturally thin as the Namuh models, even the slender women dieted—just in case. Hardly anyone felt they could relax and eat normally. Dieting became the normal thing to do! No one felt happy anymore, because they were all trying so hard to be thinner.

Now that the Namuh women felt a need for improvement in their looks, they began to buy lots of cosmetics and other products to make up their faces and color their hair, trying to hide the ways they felt imperfect. When they went shopping, instead of looking for clothing they felt would be fun to wear, they tried to fit into the clothing they saw looking great on the models. Well, I wish I could say this was as bad as it got, because things got even worse.

All those dieting Namuh women began to feel what any dieting person feels: hungry! Well, this should be no surprise, but these Namuh had lost all common sense. Hungry? They began to feel something was wrong with them when they were hungry! Can you imagine such a thing? When they had finally become so hungry from all the dieting that they couldn't stand it, you can guess what happened. What happens to any creature that is so hungry? When they would finally let themselves eat, planning, of course, to eat just a little, they couldn't stop—not for a long time and not until well after they were quite stuffed.

Now you would think they would understand this is the natural thing to do, wouldn't you? Of course, anyone would have to eat, and eat and eat after getting so hungry—don't you agree?

But they did not understand this. Instead, they felt horrible about having eaten so much. They decided it meant they should try to diet more and be even stricter about it. Because by now, most blamed themselves. They believed their hunger was the problem. They felt like gluttons around food and thought their overeating proved it. They did not stop to think anyone would be extra hungry if they didn't eat enough. So back to dieting they went.

Well, guess what? They did so much dieting and so much overeating to make up for it that many of them overate themselves right into larger and larger sizes. The thinner they tried to be, the fatter they got! The ones who didn't get fat— well, they were still afraid food would make them get fat. Everyone was miserable.

One day the Namuh women—who had been so busy feeling bad and comparing themselves to the models and to each other that they had almost forgotten how to talk to each other—started talking. Not about their diets or how fat they felt, but *really* talking about how unhappy they were. They asked, "Is this how it is supposed to be when you grow up?" They missed how it was when they were children. Some could recall when they simply ate plenty of good food and then went out to play. They remembered they had felt so satisfied after eating, they could go until the next meal without being hungry! They noticed the photos hanging in the houses of their parents and grandparents and aunts and uncles.

They realized that these grown-ups were all different sizes and shapes and had many, many different looks and styles.

They said, have you noticed that every kind of animal in the world is so cute when it's young? Whenever anyone looks at kittens or puppies—even little boys—they ooh and aah. But when little animals or little boys grow up, their looks change. Those cute little ones don't just get taller, they get fuller; they fill out. While some are still good-looking, we don't ooh and aah at them anymore. Most simply look average—not beautiful or ugly. We love them just the same.

They asked, why are we all trying to keep on looking like puppies and kittens and young monkeys? It's time for us to look like who we were meant to be. Namuh are born to be all different sizes and shapes—big, small, round and soft; with shapes like pears, apples, or carrots, or willow trees; muscled or dainty; short and tall; with imperfect faces to top it all!

The Namuh females decided it was not worth it to spend their lives feeling bad because they could not be something they were not meant to be. Now, just as they had never felt bad not being rich or famous—because they had not expected it of themselves—they came to understand that to be happy they should not expect to look other than who they were born to be.

Finally they realized what they had tried to do could not work. Finally, they could stop feeling like failures! Instead they could be free to become the best they could be in all ways, enjoying the bodies they were born to have.

They dressed and decorated themselves their own special ways, understanding that Namuh could look attractive in lots of different ways. They bought things they needed or liked, rather than in the hopes of looking like the models. They ate lots of different foods until they were full, and then they went on to play, work, and school. In the end, the advertisers weren't quite so rich. But they had not meant to cause such harm. They were glad that everyone was happier, content to be who they were.

TALKING WITH KIDS

After reading the story be sure to talk about it. Ask your child what she thinks about how the Namuh women came to feel about themselves. Why does she think this happened? Does she think this could happen in our country? Can she imagine starting to feel the way the Namuh girls and women felt? Can you? Have either of you ever known anyone who seemed preoccupied with food and hunger all the time? Were they on a diet, or feeling they *should* be on a diet? How did your child feel when the Namuh women realized how unhappy they were trying to be something that they could not be? Can you think of a time when this happened to you or to your child? How did that feel, and what did you or she do? Don't forget to see if your child can figure out why the author called these people the Namuh.

You will find many opportunities to refer back to this story in casual conversations with your children in everyday life. For example, when you spot photos of typical fashion models in magazines or store windows at the mall, comment on the lean, lanky (or downright skinny) look they all share. You can say, "I wish those advertisers would show models that look like *real* people!" When, on occasion, you see a "normal" size model, this is a great chance to praise that advertiser. Keep it light. You can say "Whew! What a relief!" If you overhear someone saying she "feels fat" or "needs to go on a diet," you can ask, "Does that sound like the Namuh?" Don't overdo it, but the innumerable advertisements for unhealthy weight-loss diets that bombard us every day can serve as great reminders of what happened when the Namuh restricted their eating. There may be someone in your family or circle of friends who has "dieted themselves into larger and larger sizes" (perhaps even you). If you take care not to violate anyone's privacy and speak the truth with kindness and compassion, disclosing this basis for someone's overweight status or obesity can be a powerful lesson. After reading the lessons that follow, you will be even better equipped to speak in a helpful way to your child about today's image consciousness, eating, and weight-related problems. And to explain that it doesn't have to be this way!

BODY LIFT
FAMILY PORTRAIT

The Namuh is, in part, a story of a people who hung portraits on their walls. Suggest that your child draw a picture of two or more friends or family members whose portrait she or he might like to see on your wall. Help your child think of people who are different sizes and shapes by referring to this line in the story: "big, small, round and soft; with shapes like pears, apples, or carrots, or willow trees; muscled or dainty; short and tall; with imperfect faces to top it all!"

BODY-ESTEEM AFFIRMATIONS

When your child has learned the essential message of this lesson, she will understand or relate to affirmations like these:

- Sometimes groups of people can learn to value beliefs and behaviors that do not make them happy.

- I know that looks make a first impression, but what is most important is often not seen right away.
- I can admire beautiful or handsome people without feeling I should try to imitate them.
- I know I do not need to be slim or "beautiful" to be attractive and desirable.
- It might be nice to have a different look, but I accept myself for who I am.
- People are born to be many different sizes and shapes.

Lesson 2:
We Are More Than How We Look

"Looks are everything. If you don't have
the right look, you might as well not even
go to school." —Natalie, age thirteen

Natalie's shocking words reflect the feelings of far too many of
her peers across the nation. By fifth or sixth grade, the excessive
emphasis on appearance places an extreme burden on most of
America's girls, along with a growing number of boys. A few
young people have even told me they began to feel the pressure
to have the "right" look as early as second or third grade.

Insecurity about appearance is bad enough, but children
also learn from an early age that they should *act as if* they are
not troubled by self-conscious insecurity. Many readers have
probably had firsthand experience with this split between the
"real me" and the public persona who presents to the world
what we believe the world wants to see. This disconnect from
our true selves reflects an erosion of body and self-esteem
that is damaging at any age, but is especially so in children.
When we carefully watch the appearance, actions, and voices
of children, it is startling to imagine that underneath their
laughter, they may already feel anxious about how they look.

Healthy body esteem, along with its counterpart, self-esteem,
is based on appreciation of inner qualities and skills that make
us competent, loveable, and ultimately, human. But what happens to self-esteem when playground lessons teach our kids that
there is a short list of criteria determining what it takes to be
"in" and a fine line that keeps kids "out." What if inner beauty
isn't on the list of criteria? Inner beauty may become a worthless

cliché to kids who just want to be included, but who learn that the "right" external appearance is the necessary ticket.

Whether your child is a natural beauty according to today's external standards, an average, ordinary-looking kid, or unique in her appearance, it is unlikely she or he will be immune from this strain. Maintaining a sense of identity that is based on substance rather than superficial appearance is hard when the "image is everything" myth is presented as real. As parents, our job is a challenge: to help our children minimize this struggle and to prevent worries about appearance from growing into a "looks are everything" mentality. This lesson will help you reinforce your child's sense of herself as a whole person who is more than the sum of her body parts—in spite of messages from the outside world.

BE HONEST—LOOKS DO MATTER

In our desire to counterbalance the overemphasis on looks that has consumed our culture, we may be tempted to tell kids that looks don't matter at all. But to suggest that looks are "not important," *especially* in today's world, is false, and our kids will spot this a mile away. They'll rightly decide we aren't to be trusted on this subject. It's critical not to lie to kids about the role of looks. What can we do instead?

We could try to convince our children that they *are* physically beautiful or handsome with a continuous stream of compliments. Unfortunately, relentless compliments only reinforce that how they look *is* very important. And what do we say to the many pubescent children who look somewhat awkward and out of proportion in their appearance, are plain, or do not have the perfectly symmetrical features that most would consider "beautiful"?

I can attest to the fact that simply ignoring looks entirely is not the answer. When my daughter was in the sixth grade, I had been writing and testing my *Healthy Body Image* curriculum for two years. She was the guinea pig for many of the activities I developed, and I had purposefully avoided comments on her outward appearance, instead emphasizing inner qualities. But I cringed the day she told me she didn't know I thought she was beautiful—certainly not the outcome I had intended! A long talk about her glorious eyes, heart-melting smile, olive skin, and delightfully curly hair followed immediately.

Looks do matter. It misses the point to pretend that they do not. For the most part, we cannot help ourselves from looking and from liking or not liking what we see—a little more, a little less. We have our preferences. Looks are what we meet first in a face-to-face encounter, and what we see does affect us—at least until we have a voice, words, a facial expression, a gesture to add to our first impression. Looks matter more to the young, but can make a difference to all of us throughout life. Biases about looks result in people being chosen or not chosen, from the playground to the boardroom. Jobs, mates, friends, sales, service, and attention are sometimes won or lost because of how we look. Prejudices exist, and we should not pretend to our children that they don't. Prejudicial attitudes are wrong, but they are reality. As such, kids need help to learn how they will manage their lives in the face of these attitudes. "Ideally" beautiful children, plain children, physically awkward children, skinny children, fat children, very tall children, midgets, scarred and misshapen children—*all* will be superficially judged and will judge themselves on the basis of their looks. The question is not *whether* this will happen. The question is how in balance or out of balance the judgment will be. Is it possible to keep the *relative* value of appearance in perspective?

Children who are very young or who have not yet been brainwashed by the culture seem to innately know how to do this. In a discussion of the *Healthy Body Image* curriculum, one fifth-grade girl said:

> *I know that I'm not that much of a great looking person. But it really doesn't matter to me because I know that looks are just one thing, and I think there are a lot of other great things about me. I know some people who are really good looking and even though people make a big deal about how beautiful they are, I don't think they are any happier than I am. In fact, it seems like some of them are always running to the bathroom to comb their hair or something. I'm glad I don't worry about how I look all the time.*

The director of a private elementary school in Manhattan told me she always made it a point to greet students each morning as they arrived at the school door. She was startled to realize one day that the vast majority of her comments to young female students pertained to how nice they looked, while comments to boys were of another nature. All of a sudden she began to think about the impact of this message. She decided to balance her comments, reinforcing various aspects of her students' personalities, talents, skills, and beauty that were not external. The following conversation tips and activities will help both you and your children to identify many different parts of their identity to reinforce as they grow up.

TALKING WITH KIDS

Formulas for feeling good and bad

Ask your child to think of something she does okay but is not great at.

Now ask her to think of someone who is an expert at that activity.

Finally ask your child to imagine how she would feel about herself if she had to compete against the expert, and the *only* thing that would be judged was that one skill. This, of course, would be a *formula for feeling bad.* Here are two examples of formulas for feeling bad. Use these or your own real-life scenarios to help your child understand how such a formula works.

- Maybe you love to play tennis, but are average at best. Imagine playing in front of an audience against a champion tennis player who won't let up. You're barely in the game. By the end of the match, you feel awful about yourself.

- Maybe you love to bake, but imagine yourself bringing your humble cake to the home of a world-class pastry chef, whose table is loaded with amazing desserts. You feel as inferior as your cake looks compared to the chef's masterpieces.

When we feel bad, often it's because we are comparing ourselves against a standard that is not realistic for us, and we have forgotten who we are. In the story of the Namuh, the women became unhappy when they compared themselves to images of models. This was not realistic for most of them. They also compared only one part of themselves: their looks. Could anyone feel good with this formula?

Another child-friendly example would be: *A banana wishing it could taste like an apple = one sad banana!* See if your child can think of a time in her own life when she has experienced a formula for feeling bad.

In addition to being careful

Too much focus on one attribute at the expense of others can place a person at risk for unhealthy attitudes and behaviors.

about who we compare ourselves to, remembering all the many parts of who we are is a safeguard against feeling bad. Try not to focus too much attention on any one part. Explain to your child that sometimes when people grow up, they start to care too much about one aspect of themselves: looks. This can lead them to forget that there is much more to them than appearance, and they become unhappy.

How important are looks?

As we get older, we may want to wear certain clothes that we like or that express something about us, like "I'm a hockey fan" or "I went to dance camp." We learn that a friendly smile can say, "I hope you want to get to know me." It is a safe bet that *everyone* wants to look appealing. We all need people, and how we look on the outside is *one part* of what attracts us to each other.

How important are good looks? Here are some questions to help your child think about this:

- Are good looks as important as being smart, having a sense of humor, or being a kind person?
- Are they as important as caring about others or taking care of the earth?
- Are good looks as important as good health, being a good athlete, or being a good citizen?
- If you had to choose, would you rather have good looks or an interesting, well-paying job?
- Do we need good looks to be liked? Why, or why not?
- Finally, who decides who or what is "good-looking" and how is it decided? (Also see lesson 9.)

STACKING THE DECK

Looks are one part of who we are. But the more we remember all the different parts of who we are, the stronger we will be. Pull out an old deck of playing cards that you do not mind destroying, or any stack of paper that is too thick to tear when it is stacked together. Tell your child that each card or page represents one of her many qualities or parts. Ask her if she can tear any one or even two stacked cards or pages in half (which she will easily do). Then put all the cards or pages in a stack. Ask her if she can tear the stack of cards when they are all together. (Be sure you have enough so it cannot be done.)

Like this whole deck of cards, the more we are mindful of all of the many parts of our whole self, the stronger we are. To be as strong as we can be, it is important to recognize and acknowledge all the many parts that make us a whole person—a whole boy or a whole girl. This is a *formula for feeling good.*

BODY LIFT
THE BALANCED IDENTITY MOBILE

Building an Identity Mobile will demonstrate to your child how important it is to have a balanced sense of ourselves. If there isn't time for or interest in building the mobile, it will still be very valuable for your child to complete the Identity Survey that follows. Children like this activity because it is all about them, but it is even more fun if you and/or others in the family do it with them as well. The survey will be used later to create the Identity Mobile. (You may photocopy it for use with more than one child.)

YOUR IDENTITY SURVEY:
MANY PARTS MAKE YOU STRONG

Check all the things you think are part of you, including

- All of the things you enjoy doing, whether or not you do them well
- All of the things you can do well, even if you do not enjoy them or do them often
- All of the things you have never tried, but want to try in the future

I am physically active.

_____ I run.

_____ I throw.

_____ I catch things (for example, a ball or Frisbee).

_____ I have lots of energy to be active for a long time.

_____ I lift heavy things.

_____ I climb.

_____ I jump.

_____ I dance.

Sports:

_____ I ski.

_____ I skate.

_____ I swim.

_____ I ride a bike.

_____ I do gymnastics.

_____ I wrestle.

_____ I play basketball.

_____ I play tennis.

_____ I play football.

_____ I play soccer.

_____ I ride horses.

_____ I play volleyball.

_____ I run track or jump hurdles.

_____ I play hockey.

List other physical activities or specific sports that are part of who you are: _____

_____

I am creative or artistic.

_____ I am artistic. (In what way?) _____

_____ I write poetry or stories.

_____ I participate in theater productions.

_____ I dance.

_____ I sew.

_____ I build things or do crafts. (What kind?) _____

_____ I am musical. (In what ways?) _____

List other creative or artistic abilities: _____

_____

I have intelligence.

I do

_____ Math

_____ Spelling

_____ Foreign languages

_____ Science

_____ Reading

_____ Writing
_____ Creative problem solving

I learn new things.

_____ I try new things.
_____ I learn from mistakes.
_____ I am willing to try things I might not be successful at.
_____ If something is hard, I keep at it.
_____ I finish projects or assignments.

I am a good citizen (part of my community).

_____ I am respectful.
_____ I pitch in to help.
_____ I am responsible.
_____ I am compassionate (caring).
_____ I participate. I do my part.
_____ I take care of the environment.
_____ I try to think about what is best for everyone.

I have relationships.

_____ I like people.
_____ I am kind of shy.
_____ I am outgoing.
_____ People can count on me.
_____ I feel love for someone.
_____ I am kind.
_____ I include people who are not my best friends.
_____ I like to laugh with people.
_____ I am interested in lots of things.

_____ I am a team player. I do what I'm asked for the sake of the team.

_____ I can be a leader. I can take charge when needed.

_____ I can laugh at myself and at my mistakes.

_____ I care about how people feel.

_____ I can resolve conflicts.

_____ I am fun to be with.

_____ I have a sense of humor.

_____ I like to help others.

_____ I am polite.

_____ I can be serious.

_____ I am a good listener.

_____ I share with others.

I take pride in my appearance.

_____ I like to wear my hair a certain way.

_____ I keep myself clean.

_____ I like to wear my favorite colors.

_____ I like clothes that say something about me.

_____ I like to wear hats, jewelry, or other accessories.

_____ I like to look friendly or inviting to people.

_____ I like my color of hair.

_____ I like my eyes.

_____ I like my skin coloring.

_____ My hair is _____ curly _____ straight.

_____ My overall size for my age is _____ bigger _____ smaller _____ average.

Another thing about my looks is _____

_____

I manage my health and keep things in balance.

____ I shower or bathe on a regular basis.

____ I eat healthy food.

____ I am physically active.

____ I play safe and smart. I take reasonable risks.

____ I stop and think about making healthy choices.

____ I know what I need deep down and can ask for it when I need to.

____ I have people who care about me, keep me company, and support me.

____ I organize and manage my time.

____ I balance work with time to relax.

____ I have realistic expectations of myself. I do my best, but don't have to do everything perfectly.

____ I can accept it when things don't work out.

____ I organize and manage my things.

____ I am able to make decisions.

____ I can say no and disagree if I need to.

I have many feelings.

Sometimes I feel

____ Happy or content

____ Sad

____ Afraid

____ Hurt

____ Angry

____ Excited

I have other interests. (Add as many as you like!)

____ I collect things. (List things you collect.) _____

____ I have a pet. (What kind?) _____

_____ I play games.

_____ I read.

_____ I play miniature golf.

_____ I do magic.

_____ I go snorkeling.

_____ I cook food.

_____ I use a computer.

_____ I have a pen pal.

_____ I build models. (What kind?) _____

_____ I build other things. (What?) _____

List other hobbies or interests: _____

_____

I have values or beliefs about life.

_____ I practice a religion. (What is it called?) _____

_____ I have a strong cultural or ethnic identity. (Which one?)

_____

A few of the most important things I strongly value or believe in: _____

_____

I have my own preferences or favorites.

List one or more for each category:

Color?

Food?

Drink?

Quiet activity?

Busy activity?

Person?

Teacher?

Animal?

Way to dress?

Memory?

Hobby?

Sport?

Fruit?

Vegetable?

Subject in school?

Song?

TV show?

Game?

Time of day?

Book?

Movie?

MAKING THE IDENTITY MOBILE

For each Identity Mobile, you will need the following:

- 12 index cards
- A paper or other disposable plate (must be able to push a paper-clip wire through it)
- Paper clips
- 12 pieces of string (colored is nice) cut into 10- to 12-inch lengths
- A nail or other object to make holes for the paper clips to go through

After your child has completed the survey, she or you should write each of the statements below on the top of one of the index cards.

- I am physically active.
- I am creative or artistic.
- I have intelligence.
- I learn new things.
- I am a citizen.
- I have relationships.
- I take pride in my appearance.
- I manage my health and keep things in balance.
- I have feelings.
- I have other interests.
- I have values or beliefs about life.
- I have my own preferences or favorites.

Next, have your child choose from each category of the identity survey those characteristics that are most important to her. Make sure she chooses at least two items from each

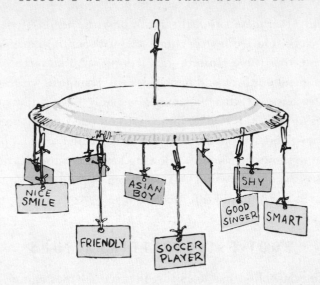

category, even if that attribute is less important to her. Then have her write her choices on the matching index card. If your child has personal attributes that don't fit into any of the categories listed, simply make additional cards, as needed.

Guide your child in constructing the mobile, using the diagram as a model. Make sure the index cards are evenly spaced around the perimeter of the plate so the mobile will balance correctly. The mobile offers the opportunity to actually demonstrate the importance of attention to all parts of ourselves in order to maintain balance and perspective. If your child prefers, she can make a balanced collage with the index cards, adding photos and pictures from magazines that reflect her interests and unique personality.

FOLLOW-UP

We all want others to know different sides of our identity. Have your child share her Identity Mobile with you in detail, as well as with other members of the family or with friends. Mom and Dad can do one too and keep them all on display. You may want to note that some parts of our identity will stay the same throughout our lives, and some parts will change as we grow.

Demonstrate what happens if we only have a few attributes in view. Lift the attribute cards on one side of the mobile to demonstrate the tilt that occurs, and then replace them to show the balance. Knowing and balancing the many parts of who you are will keep you from tipping over. Balance helps us resist formulas for feeling bad.

BODY-ESTEEM AFFIRMATIONS

When your child has learned the essential message of this lesson, she will strongly relate to affirmations like the ones below:

- How I look is part of me, but there are many important parts to who I am.
- Who I am on the inside is more important than how I look on the outside.
- I can do a lot of things.
- I have a lot to offer.
- I am strongest when I remember all aspects of my identity.
- There are some things about me I can change or improve.
- There are some things I was born with, and they will always be part of me.
- My worth cannot be measured in comparison to anyone else.
- My worth does not depend on my looks.
- I am someone who is worth getting to know.

Lesson 3:
Our Genetic Legacy

Most children today incorrectly learn that any body that is not slim is *over* the weight that it should be, that all fatness is bad, and that fatness inevitably occurs as a result of doing something wrong. The assumption that "fat people" (a label often applied to anyone with any degree of fatness) would not be the way they are (fat) if they would just eat right and exercise is deeply embedded in the contemporary American psyche. This bias holds whether a person "could stand to lose five pounds," is moderately "overweight," or is obese. This prejudice is applied even when we are completely ignorant of the actual eating behaviors or level of physical activity of a fatter person. The faulty story line is, if you are fatter than our culture's preferred look, you have only yourself to blame. Across the board, most American children who do not have the "right" (lean) body type learn to feel ashamed about what they perceive to be their "failure." Those who are naturally slim learn from an early age to anxiously scrutinize their bodies, sure that a watchful vigilance is necessary to prevent their own body's expansion.

Given the unhappiness this causes, it is high time we educate our children about the biology of body size and shape, as well as the limits to healthy size and weight "control." Children should understand from the get-go that the greatest influence for diverse body sizes and shapes is built in to their bodies before they are even born. With reasonable care, their bodies will grow in their own unique way, entirely independent of watchful external "management." Of course, reasonable care is a critical part of this formula and the topic of lessons 7 and 8. Nonetheless, the degree to which eating and physical-activity habits will *show* themselves to the outside world in the form of a fatter or thinner body is limited tremendously by our genetic inheritance. This lesson will help you teach your child that our bodies are a biological continuation of our parents' bodies, transferred through their genes. Their genes will direct their body to maintain a body shape and weight range that is right for them.

WHAT ACCOUNTS FOR BIOLOGICAL DIVERSITY IN SIZE?

When babies are conceived, they are programmed to grow according to their own internal plan. Each receives twenty-three chromosomes inherited from Dad through his sperm, and twenty-three from Mom through her egg. In this way, forty-six chromosomes, or twenty-three chromosome pairs, are united to carry on the legacy of two families. The purpose of the chromosome pairs is to carry the 30,000 or so genes donated from each parent. Each and every gene contains instructions for the growth and development of a new person through infancy, childhood, adolescence, and the entire life cycle.

Genes are made of an amazing compound called DNA. DNA can be thought of as a kind of recipe book for how all the different genes should link together to result in a final product: one whole human being. Just to give you an idea of the possibilities, it has been estimated that in humans, a complete set of chromosomes contains 6,000,000,000 base pairs of DNA (six billion!), each containing a unique code for linking genes. Clearly the number of possible variations for diversity within the human species is astonishing.

Given all of the possible combinations, how is it that an individual ends up with Dad's blue eyes versus Mom's brown, or with Grandpa's curly red hair versus Mom's or Dad's straight brown hair? Why do you have your mother's pear-shaped body and your dad's short legs, while your sister is a beanpole (or vice versa)? If you want to brush up on how certain traits are passed from parents to children, including the percentage chance that one trait will be inherited over another, you can find more information in an elementary biology text at your library. But to help your child understand why kids come in all sizes, it is only necessary that you learn a few simple facts about what exactly is inherited, versus what may be influenced by eating and activity.

WHAT IS INHERITED?

Bone structure

We may or may not appreciate our height, our long or short fingers, our square or recessed jaw, but most of us learn to live with our basic frame, accepting that bones are not something over which we have any external control. Broad or narrow shoulders, wide or narrow pelvis, bowlegged or knock-kneed, a long or short waist—we do what we can with what we have. Yes, people do reshape noses or chins through cosmetic surgery, but even surgical options are very limited and far too expensive for most people to seriously consider. The size and shape of our bones is an inheritance we can do nothing about through any natural means.

Fat-to-lean body-tissue composition, location of fat stores, and base metabolic rate

Rationally, most of us know that no amount of dieting and exercising will ever make us look like supermodel Kate Moss.

At the same time, Kate Moss should know there is virtually nothing she could do to look like Olympic soccer star Mia Hamm. Even the most intensive workout program will turn very few men into Arnold Schwarzenegger look-alikes, and many who idolize Oprah Winfrey and Rosie O'Donnell will have to settle for a leaner look than that presented by these famous entertainers. Even so, a constant stream of messages reminding us of the relationship between eating, physical activity, and weight have systematically brainwashed us into forgetting that these important behaviors are only *part* of a complex formula that determines weight and shape. In fact, all bodies have a powerful genetic predisposition for fat-to-lean tissue composition, the locations where fat will be stored, and the base rate at which our bodies will use the calories we eat (metabolism).

The diverse results of this can be seen in three very broad categories of innate (built-in) body types that generally describe most people pretty well. Keep in mind that very few people fit perfectly into one category. Most of us fall somewhere in between.

Ectomorphs are born to be thin. These people have not only low body fat percentages but also a relatively low amount of muscle mass and small muscle size. Even when eating what might be considered a lot and working out aggressively, a fast metabolic rate ensures that pure ectomorphs will not gain much weight or muscle mass. This body type is naturally seen in long-distance athletes and high-fashion models. Ectomorphs tend to be small boned as well as small muscled.

Mesomorphs tend to have a low to medium body-fat percentage, along with significant muscle mass and muscle size.

Usually of average weight, mesomorphs can build muscle easily and also may lose or gain weight relatively easily up to a point or within a limited range. Their rate of metabolism adjusts readily to defend an average weight, and it's hard for them to become either very skinny or truly fat. Generally their shoulders are wider than their hips, and bones are medium to large. The pure form of this body type is naturally seen in power athletes (as opposed to long-distance athletes).

Endomorphs have a higher body-fat ratio, as well as less muscle mass and smaller muscle size. Regardless of appetite or activity level, people with this body type tend to metabolize food more slowly, gain weight easily, and be curvier than other body types. There is also resistance to losing weight, even when food intake is limited and activity is increased. Often this body type is pear shaped, with hip bones wider than shoulders. Overall bone size tends to be larger.

It is not possible to change our inherited body type. Ignorance or denial of this fact is one of the roots of most body-image and eating problems. People will argue that with sufficient calorie loading or restriction and hours of intense workouts, bodies can be forced to either build up or reduce to a size that is reminiscent of another body type. This is true in some cases. For example, a pure endomorph might temporarily approach the appearance of a mesomorph with enough effort in reducing and burning calories. But the extreme amount of time, effort, and disconnection from inner cues it would take to maintain a very slim body is virtually impossible for most people.

Many readers of this book may face battles with their own bodies. As parents, we hope to prevent our kids from engaging in this war. Information about genetic inheritance should be common knowledge for them. When kids understand their biological nature, they will understand there are limits to the degree to which they can expect to healthily control their outer packaging. Then, just as they learn to live with their diverse bone structure, eye and skin color, freckles, and certain talents, they will learn to accept their body type for what it is. When pressed to idealize one "right" body type, understanding of the genetic basis of size diversity will help our kids say, *"Get real!"* They will be ready to spend their energy instead on the positive, effective choices that will help them to be strong, well-fed, fit, and confident—inside and out, at any size.

Avoid conclusions about the size and shape of a growing child's body until he or she is fully grown. Whether a child is destined to be taller, shorter, fatter, or thinner, their natural, healthy, predisposed adult size and shape may not be apparent until they are in their late teen years.

A final reminder will relieve the anxiety of readers who are worried that teaching children about the genetic limits to body size and shape will lead them to ignore eating wisely and staying fit. The basis for this concern is understandable, since the number one reason given by Americans for healthy eating and physical activity is to reshape our bodies! But remember that this unfortunate perspective has become the norm only since children have come to believe that food intake and activity levels *alone* "control" weight and that achieving the "right" weight is critical for social acceptability. Learning about genetic influence is corrective of a missing portion of the body-size formula, not an either/or proposition. It is equally essential that your children learn that, given our innate bodies, positive lifestyle choices are the key to health and body esteem.

Lessons 7 and 8 will help you teach your child that a healthy weight depends on sound nutrition and staying in shape.

TEACHABLE MOMENTS

You can begin to teach this lesson about genetic predisposition of body size and shape as soon as your children are old enough to understand that their bodies came from their parents. Any situation in which children are observing body-size diversity offers a chance to point out in a matter-of-fact way that bodies naturally occur in all different sizes and shapes, with an endless multiplicity of other physical characteristics. Opportunities for this probably exist within your immediate family. Likewise, if you are in a situation in which prejudicial ideas are expressed—that one body shape is "good" and any other is "not good" or "bad"—you can firmly educate children about body-shape diversity.

Contrary to what you may think, it is not necessary or a good idea to try to talk children out of their preferences about size. Preferences are not necessarily the same thing as judgments and, in fact, are a part of our individuality. For example, I personally prefer chicken over fish, peaches over apples, violets over roses, and dark eyes and hair over blue-eyed blondes. But I never feel any need to belittle the alternatives. I trust that you, on the other hand, can be partial to fish, apples, roses, and blue-eyed blondes without any need to put down my favorites. Our strong tastes for this or that may even be inborn, which calls for our respect as much as any other unique, innate characteristic. Preferences make us interesting and are not, in themselves, prejudicial. Preferences (especially those that are learned and culturally reinforced) become prejudicial, and therefore dangerous, if judgments enter the picture. This is cause for concern and education.

As long as your child simply expresses a preference for a certain body look (probably this will be the lean "ideal" in today's culture), you do not need to express anything other than interest. Even so, it is important to use this opportunity to be sure your child knows she may or may not be able to have the body he or she prefers, no matter how hard she tries, if the cards weren't dealt that way. Believe it or not, this does not have to be all that painful. When people understand from the get-go what is and what is not within their reach, they ordinarily know where to put their energy. We don't usually fight with the nonnegotiables of life. You can point this out to your child, using bone structure as an example. In fact, if there is some part of your bone structure that you would prefer were different—shortness or tallness, foot size, or the shape of your hands—admit it, while noting that for the most part you spend little time feeling bad about this and certainly don't spend time, energy, money, and self-esteem trying to change it. With the givens of life, we move on pretty quickly, directing our attention to finding success with more achievable goals.

Your child will be exposed to diverse body sizes daily and to other people's judgments of those sizes as well (including propaganda about "cures" for the "wrong" body via diet advertisements). In time your child will probably demonstrate his or her personal preferences (and perhaps prejudicial judgments) about bodies. These occasions are your best opportunities for teaching your child about genetic influence and what is and is not within their control when it comes to body size and shape.

TALKING WITH KIDS

Two peas in a pod

Has your child ever been told she looks like you or another relative? If not, help her to think of two or more people, related by blood, who resemble each other in appearance. You could also find a photo in a magazine of a mother-daughter look-alike pair or of two siblings. Ask your child if she knows how people in the same family can end up looking like each other, or having similar talents. Then be sure she understands the basic information in the following paragraphs.

Genetic programming and video science

Do your children know that a VCR can be *programmed* to turn itself on, tape a TV show they don't want to miss, turn itself off, and have the tape ready when they want to watch it? If your kids know how this is done, they know that when something is programmed, it is set up ahead of time in a way that *predetermines* what it will do later. The child-friendly language that follows may help you put ideas into words easily.

In our bodies, we all have tiny genes, far too small to see, that work a lot like programming in a VCR. Many thousands of genes are passed on to us by our birthparents. These genes contain a program that tells our body when to grow, how to grow, and when to stop growing—just like the program in a VCR directs the recording of a favorite show. No one gets to choose or customize his or her own programming. It's all built in from the start, based on the genes we inherited from our parents, our parents' parents, and our parents' parents' parents. Everybody who has ever lived has a genetic program. Genetic program-ming is simply not in our control.

It's important to understand that how we look is first and foremost determined by our genes. This includes our facial fea-tures; our hair, eye, and skin coloring; how tall or short we are; how long, short, or wide our fingers, toes, and feet are; and the overall bone structure, muscles, and fat stores that provide the size and shape for our bodies. The study of genetics can be com-plicated, but the basic facts are simple: We inherit the genes that program our body's growth from our mother and father. For example:

- *You might inherit your long or short legs from either parent.*
- *You might get your hair color from your mother, but its curliness from your father.*
- *You could inherit your facial features from one parent and your musical talent from the other.*
- *Genes can skip a generation. You might inherit a talent or trait from a gene that your parents carry, but that neither has themselves. They may have passed it on to you from a grandparent, or a great-grandparent.*

Emphasize to your child that genes strongly influence not only height, but also overall body shape and weight, includ-ing fatness and thinness. Ask your child to think about and name some obvious inherited traits in her or your biological family to engage her in dialogue. If your child is adopted or not acquainted with her biological relatives, comment on the look-alike family members of friends and neighbors (or even inherited characteristics in the offspring of your pets!) to point out evidence of the transfer of genes from one genera-tion to the next.

MORE TALKING WITH KIDS

Read or paraphrase the following additional information to your child.

Many people believe the main thing that influences how big or small, fat or thin a person is, is what they eat and how much they exercise. These definitely do influence our size. Even so, more influence comes from our genes.

No matter how much we eat or are physically active, our genes will determine

1. How long, short, thick, narrow, or wide our bones will be.

Bones are the frame for our body. Bones determine height, but also how wide our shoulders and hips are, how long our back is compared to how long our legs are, how long our fingers and arms are, etc. We could have long legs, short arms, wide feet, and narrow hips, or just the opposite. It all depends on the genes we inherit. Bones also shape our face—our nose, our cheeks, and the shape of our heads.

2. Whether we are or will be generally more, medium, or less fat.

This might mean we are thinner or fatter overall, or only some parts of our bodies are thinner or fatter than the rest of our body. Almost any combination is possible (examples: fatter thighs but smaller breasts, fatter waist but thinner hips, plumper cheeks but thinner calves).

There are more normal body sizes and shapes and looks than anyone can imagine, with thousands of genes to inherit and millions, even billions of combinations. Over the next few days, notice how varied a range of body sizes and shapes exist in the world. How could there be just one—or even a few—"right" ways to look?

BODY LIFT

PICTORIAL FAMILY TREE

Guide your children in creating a family tree, going back to their grandparents' generation or even before. On a large sheet of paper, have them draw and color a pictorial family tree that illustrates as many physical traits of relatives as possible. For example, your child could include each person's hair, eye, and skin color, their curly or straight hair, relative body size and shape, facial features, freckles, other unique traits, or racial characteristics, as well as listing innate talents or skills such as musicality, athleticism, mathematic wizardry, or artistic ability. Try to include biological brothers and sisters, parents and grandparents—even aunts and uncles and great-grandparents. Get help from family members if you don't know these people very well.

IF CHILDREN ARE ADOPTED OR DO NOT KNOW THEIR BIOLOGICAL RELATIVES

Help your child focus less on their birthparents and more on the fact that their body did come from somewhere. They can assume many things about their genetic heritage, just like anyone else, and they do not have to feel this is a taboo subject. Have your child imagine and draw a pictorial family tree that includes characteristics their blood relatives must have had—because they themselves have those characteristics! For example, a tall, black-haired child who sings like a bird and is great at math could draw a set of birthparents, one or both of whom *must* have had the genes that carried these traits.

Keep in mind that it is not important that your child's drawings are perfectly accurate or great works of art. What is important is that her picture helps her think about the fact that her body came from somewhere. Her body carries forward the genetic code of her ancestry and, as such, is not hers to mold into whatever form she—or more likely, her environment—deems to be "desirable." In addition, be sure your child knows that until she grows into her adult body inheritance, she can only imagine the adult body shape that will emerge. Discourage children from drawing any conclusions about how they are going to look when they grow up.

BODY-ESTEEM AFFIRMATIONS

When your child has learned the essential message of this lesson, she will relate to affirmations like these:

- People are born to grow into all different sizes and shapes: short, tall, fat, and thin.
- I may be able to influence the fatness or thinness of my body, but there are limits to how much I can control or choose my shape.
- I may prefer a particular way to look, but I accept myself for who I am.

Lesson 4:
How the Body Regulates Weight

A recent television commercial portrayed two women debating whether or not squirrels worry about getting fat:

> *"All those nuts have a lot of calories."*
> *"Yeah, but at least squirrels get a lot of cardio!"*

Did nature really intend for humans to be so preoccupied with the effects of eating on body size? Our culture's frenzied obsession with achieving the "perfect" size means a self-defeating fight with Mother Nature. We seem to have lost all trust in our body's ability to regulate itself when it comes to weight.

Kids with strong body esteem and trust do not fear their bodies will betray them. They confidently enjoy healthy eating and physical fitness for the good health, wholesome appearance, and sheer pleasure they bring, rather than anxiously viewing these as something they should manipulate to control their size and shape. This lesson will help your child understand the built-in mechanisms that regulate weight. She will learn that, with reasonable care, she can trust her body to grow and maintain a weight that is right for her.

MANY FACTORS INFLUENCE WEIGHT

Many factors influence our weight at any given time. This is often misunderstood, because new discoveries about this are very recent, and accurate information is only starting to be publicized. Even many medical providers are confused today about the working definitions of *overweight* and *underweight,* as well as the causes of both. Most of us grew up believing that fatness of any amount inevitably results from lack of will-power and laziness, and that fatter people surely eat more and exercise less than people who are slim. But this does not account for those fatter people who eat very well and who are physically fitter and stronger than many of us will ever be. Certainly eating habits and exercise *do* influence weight. But simple equations such as "calories eaten minus calories burned = weight lost" or "3,500 calories = one pound of body fat gained or lost" ignore far too many factors and lead us to believe we have much more control over our weight than we do.

If you and I both go on vacation, and we both live on malts and french fries while lazing around the pool each day, the end result may be quite different for each of us. You may gain weight while I may not, or vice versa. Or we both may gain, but you may drop the added pounds without effort, while I hold on to them. People who eat like horses and never gain a pound drive people who are more susceptible to weight gain crazy! But the fact is that, even when eating and activity levels are identical, the end results are often very different. In the same vein, when genetically identical twins are raised separately, even with different eating habits and lifestyles, their weights turn out to remain remarkably similar. Why is this?

In the past ten years, there has been an urgent push for more research to better understand the ways in which bodies regulate weight, especially since the World Health Organization classified obesity as a global epidemic. One outcome of these new investigations is a new phrase coined by scientists to describe a major cause of our wider girth: an *obesigenic environment*. An obesigenic environment is one that has an abundance of inexpensive, high-calorie "entertainment" foods readily available and that is not conducive to physical activity. Such a setting is probably familiar to most readers, as it certainly describes much of the American landscape. But easy access to treats and a couch-potato lifestyle do not explain why different individuals respond differently to identical eating and lifestyle habits. Nor does it answer why some people are so much more likely to choose inactivity and treats, while others are constantly moving and crave only vegetables. A little information about the latest research will help you to teach your child that fatness is not merely due to a lack of willpower that stems from overeating and laziness, but can also be the result of built-in factors that are outside our control.

HOW FAT IS ACCUMULATED

Let's start with the familiar formula mentioned above: the difference between calories that are eaten and calories that get used determines the amount of energy (excess calories) that will be left over and therefore stored in the body in the form of fat.

$$\begin{array}{r} \text{Calories eaten} \\ -\text{Calories used} \\ \hline \text{Excess calories to store} \end{array}$$

In the past it was assumed that everyone's body regulated weight in pretty much this same way—with the brain sending signals to the appetite that there was a need for more food whenever the body had used most of the energy from the prior feeding. If this held true, with little effort a balance would be maintained, and weight would remain stable within an "ideal" range.

The problem is, this theory doesn't reflect reality. Some people crave more food than their bodies need to use in the short or long term. Are these people "too hungry," or do they move "too little," or both? In any case, why doesn't the brain communicate more with the fat stores and send a signal to the appetite to reduce food intake when these stores are full— since it seems to do this for people who are lean?

Likewise, when a fatter person and a thinner person both eat well and exercise to the same degree, why does only one of them store excess fuel in the form of fat? Since the metabolism of lean people is known to automatically increase in response to eating, why does this not occur for everyone? If fat people eat more than thin people, they should have the fastest metabolism rates of all! Is there a dysfunction in the amount of energy fatter people use? If so, is this because they are lazy, or are there other reasons? Perhaps fatter people who move the same amount as leaner people somehow use energy more efficiently—like an energy-efficient car that gets more miles to the gallon—so that there is always more fuel in reserve.

In 1995 a major scientific breakthrough answered many of these questions. Studies demonstrated that storage of body fat is due to many internally regulated mechanisms that are outside of our control and that are different for different people. Since then, we have identified specific genes that regulate both hormonal activity and the central nervous system, which in turn affect both appetite (what and how much food is desired) and metabolism (how fast food is used). In addition, the latest research suggests that particular genetic make-up causes people to be more or less inclined toward physical activity and determines whether they receive more or less benefit from exercise than other people. So while eating and activity have an influence on an individual's degree of fatness, weight is clearly also regulated by other built-in mechanisms that vary from person to person. If we consider what we know about bodies, this is not surprising. Bodies regulate heart rate, breathing, temperature, electrolyte and fluid balances—just to name a few functions. Why wouldn't they regulate the storage of fat as well?

EACH BODY DEFENDS A SET WEIGHT RANGE

The easiest way to understand how internal weight regulation works is to compare it to the thermostat that keeps the temperature in your home relatively constant, even when outside temperatures vary. Several functions, including metabolism, appetite, and energy level fluctuate in an effort to keep weight stable, within an average range over time, even when outside factors, such as what we ate last weekend or whether we were sedentary yesterday, vary. This weight range, which our bodies are programmed to maintain, is called our set point. Rather than a single number on the scale, our set-point range may encompass a five- to fifteen-pound span.

Human bodies are designed to defend diverse set points. Set points can change significantly over the life cycle, with aging and developmental changes (such as puberty and menopause) and during or after a pregnancy or illness. Set points may also change when new medications are taken for extended periods of time, with new, extended levels of physical activity, with changes in the percentage of muscle in the body, with extreme emotional stress, and with restricted or excessive calorie intake. But most of the factors that regulate our set point are not in our control.

Overriding our set point

In the past four decades, fads and fashions have created pressures to be very thin, and fatness of any degree has come to be scorned. Many people have found themselves at war with their bodies because their set-point weight range is higher than today's body "ideal." The lower weight that so many wish for is not natural for them, which means it is not achievable through ordinary, healthy choices. Rather than accepting this limit, we try to override our internal weight regulatory system and force weight to a lower number on the scale. This requires turning away from ordinary healthy self-care to extraordinary means, such as calorie restriction or excessive exercise.

Extraordinary means can seem to be a good solution at first, but serious problems occur when we try to pull rank on the natural functions of our bodies. Unless our bodies are physiologically predisposed to a lower weight (for example, if our weight has been previously forced above our set point through excessive calories or inactivity), then weight loss virtually always meets with internal resistance. Even with enormous and continuous effort, our bodies will fight to regain the status quo. Such efforts are usually counterproductive in the long run and can even do permanent harm.

Before you can guide your child to live healthily and graciously within a natural, healthy weight, you may need to examine your own participation in the body wars and the extraordinary efforts we use to resist our biological predispositions. Do any of the examples below apply to you? If so, be easy on yourself. Billions of dollars are spent annually to make these extraordinary methods seem like they are reasonable, healthy options. Even physicians are vulnerable to such hype.

- Do you participate in the diet mania that is a normal part of life for huge numbers of Americans—sacrificing important nutrients and energy intake in an effort to drive your weight below its set point, blaming yourself when weight is regained?

- Do you dedicate hours of your daily life to exercise for the purpose of burning calories—hoping to force your body weight below your natural set point?
- Have you chosen not to take life-enhancing medications, such as antidepressants, or prednisone because weight gain (a rise in your set point) is listed as a possible side effect?
- Have you turned to surgical solutions to lower your weight for nonmedical reasons?
- Have you taken experimental diet drugs, such as fen-phen or Redux, or highly questionable over-the-counter diet supplements in order to force your weight to a lower level?
- Are you among the many who felt desperate and despairing when dangerous weight-loss drugs were removed from the market, or were no longer freely prescribed by physicians?

Once upon a time, I would have had to answer yes to the first and last two questions. I was eighteen years old when I became dependent on diet pills that were prescribed by my physician. I truly believed 123 pounds was too fat for my five-foot-four-inch frame. By the time the medical community recognized the danger and stopped writing easy prescriptions for amphetamines, I was twenty-two and terrified about how fat I would become without these appetite killers. Despite the high blood pressure they caused me at so young an age, I probably would have continued to take them indefinitely if I'd had the chance, because they "worked."

Something is wrong when so many have so much trouble accepting their body's own internal weight regulation. Our nation's obsession with forcing weight below our natural set-point range is a misguided belief that we can mess with Mother Nature—and win.

Similar problems occur when body weight is forced above

its natural set point, for example, when males go to extremes in order to "bulk up." In recent years we have seen an alarming rise in the use of dangerous drugs that trick the body into weight and muscle gain. In rare instances, females who are extremely thin by nature may try to add curves through body-building drugs and surgical implants.

Most people feel that adding excess pounds is a piece of cake. Many people wonder why bodies can be so resistant to losing weight below a set-point range, but more readily gain weight above this range. The fact that we ask this question probably reveals our denial about how unnatural the high-fat, high-sugar, supersized eating habits and sedentary lifestyles of many Americans really are. Eating for amusement and intense flavor, paired with physical inactivity, is so much a part of our lives that it has become a daily occurrence for people to eat a very large number of empty calories and not even recognize this is what they are doing. Even those who are not genetically predisposed to a fatter body frequently push beyond the upper limits of their set point when eating is viewed primarily as "entertainment" and leisure habits are primarily sedentary.

Scientists have theorized that the ease of weight gain (compared to weight loss) is a leftover survival mechanism from historical times when food was periodically scarce. This is not unreasonable, since an abundance of food and lack of need for physical exercise to get food (an obesigenic environment) are very recent events. Since our genes have not changed as rapidly as our environment, a big rise in fatness and obesity should really be no surprise. Our bodies are still wired genetically to eat a lot in times of abundance, to store as much as possible as reserve fat, and then to burn this reserve very slowly over the famine—ensuring survival of the species. For better or worse, our weight regulatory systems have no way to know that famine is no longer a threat, and a large amount of stored fat is really not necessary.

In short, bodies are genetically predisposed to be diverse in size and shape regardless of the environment—feast or famine. But in times of abundance (today's environment), those who are genetically more susceptible to gaining weight will take the most advantage of this. Natural diversity in an obesigenic environment means a much greater percentage of the population gains weight. Many scientists propose that unhealthy fatness will continue to increase regardless of our best efforts unless there is a major increase in the kind of education this book provides, as well as a decrease in marketing of low-nutrient foods and sedentary entertainment.

With reasonable care and feeding, your child can trust her body to arrive at the weight that is healthy for her without undue preoccupation or anxiety. In today's world of abundant food and sedentary entertainment, knowledge about the internal weight regulatory system will help her to respect Mother Nature, maintain body esteem, and be motivated to make positive choices.

TALKING WITH KIDS

Aside from the pure pleasure that eating brings, food in our body functions much the same as gas in our car. You can introduce this topic to your child anytime you are at the service station filling your gas tank. Keep it really simple. Tell her that gasoline is a fuel that burns very easily. When you turn the car key, a rapid series of sparks burn the gas a drop at a time. This burning creates a force that runs the engine. Does your child know what happens when a car has burned up all its gas?

Tell her that, like gas for a car or truck, the food she eats provides fuel for her body. Even though there is no actual spark or fire, food is "burned," or turned into energy, a little at a time to keep us going. Of course, there is an important difference between a car with an empty gas tank and a person with an empty stomach. See if she can name it: a car out of gas will suddenly die. In contrast, a human without food will not die, at least not right away. A human without food will feel weak and uncomfortable, but can live without food for many days or maybe even weeks. Why is this?

Nature has provided humans with wonderful safeguards: a way for our bodies to keep *reserve* energy or backup fuel in the body. This way, even if we run out of food, we can still live for quite a while. In an emergency, this reserve energy gives us time to find food and refuel ourselves.

Ask your child if she knows where the body stores its reserve fuel. Extra energy is stored in the body as fat. If you can do it in a positive, matter-of-fact way, pinch a bit of your own fat to demonstrate that you mean common, ordinary body fat. The message, of course, is that yes, you are comfortable having some fat. Then share the following information about fat storage and metabolism with your child.

The body's reserve fuel

Most of us are lucky to have plenty to eat. This is not true everywhere in the world. But with enough to eat, it can be easy to forget how important it is that the body can store reserve fuel in the form of fat. If suddenly food were not available, body fat could mean the difference between life and death. In the past, fat meant you could survive the winter (in caveman days) or that you were wealthy and had money for food (during hard times). Sometimes people think fat is just bad, but without fat storage, all cavemen and -women would have died, and we would not be here today. We should be thankful for our ability to store fat!

When people don't have to worry about starvation, they have time to think about other things. One thing well-fed people tend to think more about is looks. Fads and fashions about looks have come and gone over the years. These days, people have decided that slimness is preferred for women, and a very lean and muscular look is preferred for men. The more this look has caught on, the more fatness of any amount has come to be viewed as a bad thing, as if getting rid of it were entirely within our control, and Mother Nature had no part in it. Many people decided fat was always a sign of eating too much and being lazy. Eating and exercise can influence weight, but this explanation ignores many other causes of fatness or thinness.

Why do people store more or less fat?

What we eat and how physically active we are can influence weight, but this is not the whole story. The first reason why people store more or less fat is that each of us has a system for regulating weight that is built in to our bodies. The way this system works is inherited through our genes and has many parts, some of which are complicated to understand. One part of this system that is easy to understand is called metabolism. When you understand metabolism, you will know one of the reasons why some people store more fat than others do. Metabolism is the means by which bodies "burn" fuel, or transform the food you eat into energy to keep you going and growing—just like gas keeps your car going.

The speed at which metabolism burns the food we eat is different for everyone. Some people have a fast metabolism, which burns the food they eat very quickly. Others have a slow metabolism, which burns the food they eat much more slowly. Your speed of metabolism—fast, medium, or slow—determines how long it takes for the food you eat to be used as energy by your body. Your rate of metabolism is inherited through your genes. It is built in, and it is preset for you. When food is used slowly because of a lower metabolism, the digested food that is not yet needed for energy must be stored in your body's "reserve tank" in the form of fat.

The rate of metabolism or the amount of fat stored does not affect hunger. Soon after our stomach empties, we naturally feel hungry. There is no basis for the common belief that fatter people should be less hungry.

BODY LIFT
THE METABOLISM GAME

This activity is a discovery game for you and your child. You present a situation to your child and then raise several questions. The answers will reveal the effects of a slow, medium, and fast rate of metabolism. Be sure to give her a chance to answer each question before jumping in.

Tell your child to pretend she has five friends, all of whom just happen to be the same age and the same height. To help your child imagine these friends, draw five simple faces on a sheet of paper, referring to each one as you talk about them. She can even name them if she likes. Then describe the following scenario about these five friends to your child.

Imagine that your friends enjoy spending all their time to-gether every day, playing hard, working hard, and sometimes just hanging out. At mealtime they are all very hungry. Let's say that these friends all eat exactly the same food in the same amount every day. For example, for lunch they might have a sandwich, an apple, a pickle, some carrots, a couple of cookies, and a glass of milk. Whatever one eats, they all eat. They also get exactly the same amount of physical exercise.

Although they are a lot alike, each of these friends is also unique. Each one has a different rate of metabolism, or speed of burning the food they eat. There is no easy way to measure a person's rate of metabolism. We cannot check it, like body tem-perature. But let's say we know the following: One has a very fast rate of metabolism. One has a very slow rate of metabolism. The other three have medium rates of metabolism: a little fast, just average, and a little slow. (Assign them each a rate of me-tabolism.)

Now ask your child if the friend with a very fast rate of metabolism will burn the food energy she eats slowly or quickly. Will this have an influence on her body size and shape? Will she have a lot of fat stored or very little?

This friend will be very slim because her body burns every-thing she eats very quickly. There is rarely any need to store any unburned food energy as fat. (Draw a slim body for this friend.)

Next, have your child consider the friend with a very slow rate of metabolism. Will this friend's slow metabolism burn the food energy she eats slowly or quickly?

Slowly! It may be time to eat again before she has burned all the food energy from the last meal.

What influence will this have on her body size and shape?

This friend will naturally be somewhat fat, maybe even very fat. Even when she eats the exact same lunch as her friends, there will probably be unburned food energy that needs to be stored as fat. (Draw a round body for this friend.)

Do you think this fatness would keep this fatter friend from feeling hungry at the next mealtime?

Some people think that fatter people should not be hungry again until they burn up some of the stored fat. But this is not true. She would be just as hungry as her friends, because fatness is not stored inside her stomach. Her stomach would be empty by the next meal. Empty stomachs feel hungry to everyone in the same way, whether we are fat or thin.

Finally, have your child consider the three friends with the medium rates of metabolism. Will these friends' medium metabolism burn the food energy they eat slowly or quickly?

People with average rates of metabolism will tend to use most of the food they eat most of the time, but not all of the food all of the time. So these friends would be average—one a little fatter, one a little thinner, and one in between—not fat and not thin. An average metabolism means their bodies would naturally store some fat reserve, but not a lot. (Draw the varying body shapes for these friends—a little more, medium, and less fat.)

It is a myth that all people would be the same size and shape if everyone ate very well and exercised. All bodies need to be fed well and kept fit for the sake of health. Most normal, healthy people store some fat on their bodies—some a little, some a lot, and most are in the middle. Well-cared-for bodies will always come in many different normal sizes and shapes, not only short to tall but also thin to fat—thanks to our body's internal weight regulatory system.

BODY-ESTEEM AFFIRMATIONS

When your child understands this essential lesson, she will
embrace statements like these:

- Each person's body has built-in mechanisms that regulate
  weight.
- With good food and exercise, our bodies will burn the food
  we eat to maintain a weight that is natural for us.
- One mechanism that regulates weight is called metabolism. Each person has her own metabolic rate, which tells
  her body how fast to burn food for energy: slow, medium, or
  fast.
- Each person's rate of metabolism will determine how
  much food energy her body will use right away and how
  much will be stored as reserve energy, or fat. People with
  faster metabolism rates will burn food energy more quickly
  and will store very little. People with slower rates will burn
  food energy more slowly and will store more energy as fat.
- Because of differences in metabolism, even if we all ate
  exactly the same food and were physically active to exactly
  the same degree, we would still be different sizes and
  shapes—from short to tall, and fat to thin.
- We cannot assume from appearance alone that a thin person eats less or a fat person eats more.

Lesson 5:
Changes in Puberty

Appearance changes throughout life. This fact seems so obvious, you may wonder why kids need to be taught it. Unfortunately, with the barrage of messages urging us to "avoid weight gain forever," an increasing number of eight- and nine-year-old girls are restricting their eating in an effort to keep their prepubescent shapes.

Yet prepubescent children are on course for nature's most exciting and dramatic example of inevitable change, including a normal gain in weight and shape that occurs—sometimes very rapidly—with the transition into young women and men. Kids need our help to be ready.

This lesson will help your child understand more specifically how her size, shape, and appearance may change during this tumultuous time. Puberty naturally provokes kids' interest in looks. It's both crucial and logical then to introduce healthy, realistic expectations, attitudes, and social behaviors when their preoccupation with appearance is at its peak.

PREPARING YOURSELF

Many adults have not had the opportunity to become well informed about the expected outward physical changes that are a normal part of puberty for both boys and girls. This, coupled with our society's fat phobia, means that kids (especially girls) rarely get enthusiastic support for the entirely normal and expected rounding out and weight gain that is part of their development. Lacking facts and encouragement, girls at this tender age respond by comparing their budding bodies to the unrealistic, culturally sanctioned ideal body. Since the ideal is a body type that almost none of them will or should maintain, most normal-weight girls end up feeling bad about their healthy, growing bodies. Boys too are left to compare their bodies to societal ideals and are then often blamed for having unrealistic expectations of themselves and of the opposite sex.

Since comparisons are inevitable, our goal is to help our children to compare their bodies to what is normal, healthy, and diverse, rather than to unrealistic, unhealthy, and prejudicial ideals. This will enhance their body esteem and help them begin puberty with realistic, nonjudgmental expectations that will reinforce body esteem and encourage healthy body image.

The more at ease and confident you are about your child's physical development, the easier it will be for him or her. When my own daughter was entering this stage of life, I felt uncertain about when to bring up the body changes that lay ahead. I didn't want to impose information before she had any interest, but I didn't want her to sit with unanswered questions either. I remembered my own anguish as a fifth grader—worrying about the small lumps under my otherwise flat chest, fearing these were a malignant growth. When I finally overcame my embarrassment, I learned from my mother that these "breast buds" were nothing to worry about. I also realized that my mother's awkwardness made it too hard to ask her any more questions about my body's development.

Naturally I wanted it to be different for my daughter. I wanted to talk with her at the right time, in a comfortable mother-daughter way that encouraged her confidence in me. The problem was, I really didn't know exactly what good information should be provided, when and how to begin, and what was age appropriate.

I ended up waiting too long, which I now know is very common. While good information is good no matter when it is provided, children typically have a threshold for talking about their body's development. Before this threshold, most kids are relatively open to information that caring adults offer about their bodies, as long as it comes to them in a sincere, friendly way. After this threshold, the exact same conversation will commonly be met with eye rolls, protests of "already knowing," and embarrassed silence. For most parents, given the options of a little soon or a little late, the choice is a no-brainer: earlier is better.

Teachers of my curriculum consistently say fourth-grade girls and boys show intense interest in this topic. Children in Western countries develop physically at an earlier age than ever before, and these changes in their own and their classmates' bodies do not pass unnoticed. Many girls show visible signs of puberty by third or fourth grade—even though their classmates may not show similar growth for three to five more years. Boys in general lag somewhat behind girls in their growth spurts, and if you and they do not know this is a normal gender difference, boys may worry needlessly.

Once kids notice changes, they need information to correctly interpret what they see. If adults appear nervous, perhaps acting as if they don't notice these developments, children may think the subject is taboo. Such avoidance can contribute to shame or embarrassment about pubescent growth. You may remember from your own childhood that taboo talk is often fuel for playground gossip and teasing—which is best kept to a minimum. To prevent anxiety and self-consciousness, it's good to minimize misinformation from unreliable sources. To discourage teasing, normalize pubescent changes by offering information in a matter-of-fact way. Unless you tell them so, your children may not know they can and should ask questions freely and that sound information is available.

Some of you will find that talking with your kids about their growth in puberty is easy to do; you merely need to know *what* to convey. But if you are among the many parents who feel awkward, here are some thoughts that may help:

Will my child be embarrassed if I bring up puberty? Some parents feel anxious because they are afraid their children will be embarrassed. This could be true. At the same time, kids often take their cue from grown-ups in this regard, and their embarrassment may be a self-fulfilling prophecy in response to yours. Changes that are observed out loud in a casual, positive manner, accompanied by good information, will help children view such changes as normal, inevitable, and healthy. Your comfort will help to desensitize the words used to describe changes and will reduce any sense of taboo talk. Practice reading aloud the "Essential Information" section that begins on page 131 until the words are natural for you. When growth and developmental changes are perceived by children to be entirely normal, body esteem and self-esteem will be enhanced.

Should talking about appearance changes in puberty be paired with talking about reproduction and sex? I recommend keeping these conversations separate. Talking to your child about the changing look of puberty should *not* feel like it is sexually loaded. Discussion of the natural rounding or filling out that accompanies pubescent development is just that. Think about how you feel when talking with your child about feet outgrowing their shoes, fingers becoming long enough to reach an octave on the piano, or weight becoming heavy enough to sit safely in the front seat of a car with air bags. That kind of ease is a model for the level of comfort you want to achieve in talking about such changes as the addition of pounds, new curves and bulk, the evolution of facial bones, and added hair.

CHANGE HAPPENS

If your child embraces adventure, and is curious and eager to try anything, she may be completely enthusiastic about body changes in puberty. At the other end of the spectrum are kids who are naturally more cautious. Kids who need more preparation to be comfortable with new experiences may worry a lot about pubescent development. Most kids fall somewhere in the middle. But even children who seem ready for anything may despair if faced with changes—like weight gain—that those around them deem as "bad." It is a good idea to prepare all children for the changing look of puberty in order to normalize and desensitize it, intercept inaccurate messages, and make the transition as smooth and easy as possible.

Growth and development is not proportionate: some body parts grow faster than others. For example, feet often grow to full size first, followed by legs and arms, and later the spine and other bones. Ears and chins grow before other facial features. If children are not told, they may worry that these awkward proportions will be permanent.

TEACHABLE MOMENTS

Everyday life offers lots of opportunities to increase your child's awareness of change as unavoidable and completely natural. For example, you can point out the following:

- Changes in nature that are certain and predictable, such as day turning into night, or the change of the seasons.
- Changes that are *expected*, but that can include unpredictable details: the exact day your dog will have her puppies, a loose tooth will fall out, or the first snow will fall.

- Unexpected changes—both happy and sad: the ball team unexpectedly loses—or wins; a teacher gives a surprise quiz; your child gets sick and has to miss a party; or she finds a dollar bill.

Many wise people have suggested that it is not change, but our resistance to change that causes stress or unhappiness. There is a lot of truth in this. Change is certain and something we must accommodate every single day in order to survive, and to thrive.

As you talk with your child about the inevitability of change, be sure she identifies big and small changes that she has already adjusted to in her life. This will remind her that she has some experience in making adjustments. Then bring up changes that lie ahead—things that are expected to happen tomorrow, next summer, or in five years. This sets the stage to introduce the changes in her body that will occur as she grows from a child into a teen and, eventually, into an adult. Explain that this important growth stage has a special name: *puberty*. It is a part of growing up, a time when bodies no longer grow merely taller, but change in other ways as well. Tell her that every single healthy person goes through puberty.

It is helpful for children to know that puberty is an in-between time when they no longer have a child's body, but do not really have an adult body either. As appearance changes slowly but continually during puberty, your child's body image—or the way she feels and thinks about her body—will change too. When your child knows what to expect, she will more easily maintain body esteem, allowing changes to unfold. She will be less likely to fight against her biological nature. She will feel good about—or at the very least, unafraid of—what is happening.

ESSENTIAL INFORMATION

Here are the minimum facts all children should understand about their changing bodies:

- Everybody goes through puberty sometime. Growth involves both getting taller and filling out.

- Everyone's body changes at different times, according to an inner body clock or predetermined schedule. How and when we grow is not something anyone has control over. It is determined before birth. There is no advantage or disadvantage to when you start puberty. Whether a growth spurt starts earlier or later will not affect how big or small someone is in the end. A growth spurt means that children grow faster than normal. On average, instead of growing about two inches per year, kids may grow four inches or more per year.

- In general, girls begin pubescent development at a younger age than boys do. The average age for girls is between ten and twelve, but this may occur as early as eight and as late as fifteen. The average age for boys to enter puberty is between twelve and thirteen, but this may occur as early as nine and as late as fifteen. Since girls tend to develop sooner, it is common for girls to be taller than boys until around the age of thirteen or fourteen.

- Some parts of your child's body will grow faster, while other parts grow slower. It's different for everyone, but the usual order is
  1. Feet
  2. Arms and legs
  3. Backbone and other bones

- It is normal to gain weight by adding body fat and bone mass during puberty. In later teen years, some muscle is also gained.

About girls

- While a few girls will remain very lean, it is normal for girls to gain body fat rapidly in puberty. Some girls may gain twenty pounds or more in one year. This is the beginning of the normal, healthy rounding out of a girl's body as she grows into a young woman. Nature intended most adult women to carry more body fat and have a more rounded figure than most boys and men. This is part of a woman's special design for bearing children and should not be confused with becoming unnecessarily fat.

- At first a girl may develop a layer of fat all over under the skin. Then it will begin to be more obvious in breasts, hips, and thighs. Some girls may get rounder first and only later gain height. Others may get quite tall and thin first, later adding curves or roundness. A few girls will remain very thin and not very rounded all their lives, whether they are taller or shorter.

- Girls' pelvic bones very gradually begin to widen. This is

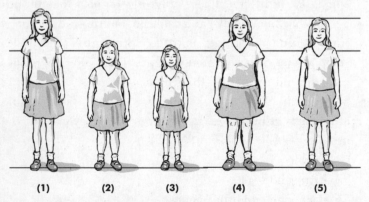

(1) Taller first, (2) Rounder first, (3) Not much taller or rounder, (4) Taller and rounder, (5) Even growth. The most common adult female shape: wider hips, narrower at the shoulders.

essential for a woman to be capable of having a baby when she is an adult.

About boys

- Once outward growth begins, boys quickly catch up. Most boys eventually become taller and more muscular than girls.
- Sometimes boys gain body fat during puberty too. Some boys become fatter before they get taller. As boys grow taller, however, they often stretch out their fatness into a taller, slimmer body. While there are natural differences, overall, most fully developed males carry less body fat than most women.
- Later in puberty, shoulders can become wider and eventually more muscular. However, boys usually do not fill out their bodies until later teen years. Then they will begin to look less like boys and more like adult males.
- More than half of all boys will have some breast swelling in puberty. This is normal and does not mean he is devel-

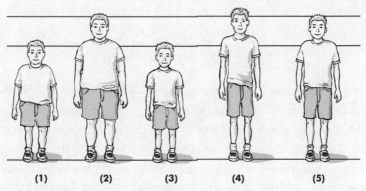

(1) Fatter first, (2) Taller and fatter, (3) Neither taller or fatter, (4) Taller, always thin, (5) Even growth. Most common adult male: broader at the shoulders than at hips.

oping breasts. It will go away in one to two years. Boys need to know not to worry about this.

- When a boy's voice box has grown larger, usually by age fourteen or fifteen, his voice becomes deeper. This may happen somewhat suddenly or in a gradual, less noticeable way. Some boys experience a cracking of their voice as they go through this change, with their voices becoming high-pitched or squeaky unexpectedly.

Other changes for both boys and girls

- Boys and girls grow hair in new places: First pubic and underarm hair, then arm and leg hair and, for boys only, eventually face and chest hair.
- Also, two glands become more active: oil and sweat. When oil glands are more active, hair gets oily faster. Also, many kids have some pimples or skin acne when they are further along in puberty. When sweat glands are more active, you may notice more perspiration, and it may have a more adult odor. When oil and sweat glands become more active, kids usually need to bathe or shower and wash their hair more often.

TALKING WITH KIDS

If a child worries that she is among the first in her age group to show signs of development, or that she is very late, help her to understand this is not "good" or "bad." Rather it's just the way that nature works sometimes. It is like the color of her eyes or how fast someone's hair grows. These things are not in our control. Of course, you should be sympathetic. In general, it is extremely difficult for children this age to be different. It would be easier if growth happened in exactly the same way and on the same schedule for everyone. But differences are a normal and necessary part of life.

It is important for your child to understand that the way one grows in puberty may not be even. For example, arms and legs may grow long, while the backbone is still short. Feet may be as big as an adult's, even two or three years before the rest of the body grows taller. Ears and chin may grow before the rest of the face. Most kids feel a little awkward or clumsy when some parts of their bodies are growing faster than other parts. Remind your child, she is not a finished product yet! That is why teasing about body changes is especially unfair and hurtful. This is not a time to judge or worry about looks. It is a time to be amazed at the many changes bodies go through as kids are growing up. Try to tell your child to relax, stay healthy, and give her body time. If she eats well, stays active, and is patient, her body will develop naturally into the size and shape it was born to be.

Because the addition of a certain amount of body fat is a natural part of puberty for all girls and many boys, it is critical to help children understand that the words *fat* or *thin* are descriptive words, not judgments. To note that a pubescent child is adding some fatness as part of their normal development should be no different from observing that his feet are growing. Take care that this is not interpreted as "getting fat," which has a negative connotation in Western culture and is routinely taken to mean we should "do something about it."

If someone teases your child about pubescent changes, you should neither panic nor ignore it. On the one hand, kids are very resilient and get through most hard knocks pretty well. On the other hand, studies have documented that teasing about body appearance can have a long-term negative effect on self-esteem. Depending on the situation, it may be sufficient to talk with your child about the ignorance that is behind teasing. If this helps your child to dismiss such comments, you can leave it at that. If your child is the victim of ongoing harassment or bullying, you will want to address this problem with other adults in charge to make sure the right message is sent and the problem is stopped.

BODY LIFT

GROWING BODIES, GROWING SKILL

Ask your child to name things her body can do now that it could not do when she was younger—along with things she will only be able to do with a more grown-up body. Suggest she draw pictures of herself doing things she enjoyed as a baby and at five years old, as well as what she enjoys now and what she will enjoy or be good at in a strong, filled-out body.

BODY-ESTEEM AFFIRMATIONS

When your child has learned the essential message of this lesson, she will relate to affirmations like these:

- There are many different, normal ways that looks can change in puberty. Most bodies get not only taller, but gain weight and fill out.
- My body's growth in puberty is not something I can or should control.
- I trust the way my body is growing.
- Boys and girls develop differently in some ways during puberty.
- It is normal for girls to gain body fat during puberty.
- Since my body will be changing over several years, I can't worry too much about how I look along the way.

Lesson 6:
Why Diets Don't Work

If someone said, "Let me tell you about my new diet," which of the following would you expect to hear about?

A. a nutritionally balanced variety of wholesome foods
B. a plan for losing weight
C. an eating plan designed to improve a medical condition, such as diabetes, heart disease, or osteoporosis

Most Americans today would choose B and associate the word *diet* with restricted food choices, hunger pangs, and willpower. While technically *diet* is defined as "the typical daily sustenance of a person or animal," this has not been the common usage of this word for several decades. Ever since pressures for a thin physique led to a preoccupation with reducing size, *diet* has become synonymous with "a plan for losing weight." According to social scientists, dieting (for weight loss) is now a "normal" eating style for women in our culture. An anthropologist would describe the typical feeding habits of modern females in the United States as characterized by anxiety about weight and the intention of reducing body size. (Actual feeding behavior may or may not fit this intention.) The definition of *ideal eating* has shifted away from "a nutritionally balanced variety of wholesome foods" to "prescribed eating for the purpose of losing weight."

If you visit a dietitian or other qualified eating specialist, you are not likely to hear the word *diet*. Eating professionals have been forced to adjust their language to avoid triggering the strong association to food restriction that the word *diet* causes in many people. In essence, the word *diet* has been taken hostage by the diet industry. It may be lost forever to the millions of "Lose Weight Fast," diet-of-the-week advertisements, books, and products, and most of us who work for a healthier approach have given up on getting it back. As a result, whether you go to a dietitian or nutritionist for a specific health or weight concern, an eating disorder, or you just want help with balanced eating, you will be guided in "healthy eating," "heart-healthy eating," "balanced eating," or "normalized eating," but *not* a "diet."

A few decades ago, I would have called the next lesson in this book "Eat a Healthy Diet." But in today's social context, the lesson is better called "Eating Well for Healthy Weight." As you read this lesson and the next, and share their messages with your children, keep in mind the popular semantics of the word *diet.* Since kids are bombarded daily with advertisements urging them to "Get the Body You Always Wanted with the New Miracle Diet!" you will want to help them distinguish between a "diet" in that context and eating well in a positive, nutritionally sound, and satisfying way.

THE PREDICTABLE RESULTS OF DIETING

Dieting came into vogue in the 1960s, even after Dr. Ansel Keys published a landmark study in 1950 that demonstrated how and why restricting hunger for weight loss backfires. While participants in this early study ate fewer than 1,000 calories per day, more-recent studies have proven that the same counterproductive results occur even with the popular, less-restrictive diets that ordinary people go on (and off) every day:

- a relentless craving for and preoccupation with food
- ravenous, overpowering hunger

- a decrease in the ability to concentrate on anything but thoughts of food
- irritability and depression
- eating far more than a normal amount to satisfy hunger when the diet ends

These symptoms of restricted eating routinely continue after the diet is stopped, even after any weight that was lost is regained. The resulting obsession and preoccupation with food contributes to long-term weight gain that is often above and beyond the original weight.

The same predictable outcomes listed above are expected to occur with *any* externally prescribed eating plan that (1) limits the amount and quality of food and (2) promises weight loss as the goal—even nutritionally balanced weight-loss plans that allow relatively satisfying portions. Sometimes parents ask, "So, what kind of weight-loss diet *is* good for my child to go on?" They don't realize this question contradicts what they just heard me say, because the answer is very difficult to take in: No weight-loss-directed diets are good.

Externally limiting food does not work primarily because humans have a built-in response that strongly resists the imposition of external controls or rules when we apply them to internally regulated vital needs. This means that even weight-loss diets that are balanced and not overly restrictive meet with resistance, if for no reason other than that the "orders" come from the outside. Consider what would happen if I told you that you must maintain an average of twelve to sixteen breaths per minute for the next hour. It doesn't matter that this is the average number of breaths that is normal for an adult person. Just receiving this prescription is likely to cause you to become very preoccupied and anxious about your breathing, especially if there are times when you need to breathe harder, such as if you have to exert yourself. Try it yourself, even for five minutes, and see what happens. Things will probably go along fine at first, but before long, one of three things is likely to happen. You will begin to hyperventilate, you will become a "compulsive over-breather," or you will begin to rigidly control all of the activities in your life in order to successfully follow my prescription. Either way, this assignment is a setup for failure, even though the prescription was not really restrictive, but rather to breathe a relatively normal amount. Of course, for those with lung disease or asthma, frustration and failure is virtually guaranteed. The rest of us might attempt to introduce periods of under-breathing—to make up for overbreathing during times of excitement or when we were in a hurry. Imagine the nation of breathing neurotics this would spawn if such behavior caught on! This may seem crazy, but it is analogous to what occurs whenever food intake is externally limited over an extended period of time. Attempts to externally "control" eating, like attempts to externally control breathing, have a very predictable, counterproductive outcome.

A second problem occurs because the goal of dieting is weight loss. It is our attachment to the belief that we can control what we cannot that backfires. As we learned in lessons 3, 4, and 5, we can certainly influence, but we cannot control body size. So, while just about anybody can achieve some weight loss by dieting, and a few people will even succeed in maintaining this loss, the result is not really in our hands. As you will recall, the outcome is strongly influenced by the internal weight regulatory system, which is primarily genetically predisposed. This is the dilemma. People may do everything "right," may stick to their diet plans—even at great emotional cost (because it does take enormous concentration and energy to eat day after day according to external rules)—but their weight may *still* not cooperate in the long run, or not as much as is desired. For these people, a prescription to diet is a prescription to fail.

In this same vein, people who might lose weight and keep it off by "diet cycling" in their teens or twenties, might or might not lose or maintain weight using the same plan in their thirties, forties, or fifties. In any case, the vast majority of people eventually go off their limited diets and regain the lost weight—often with added pounds. Our notion of weight control is clearly more of an illusion than a reality. Belief in this illusion is one of the cornerstones in the development of eating disorders, particularly anorexia. It is also a catalyst for much of the obsessive-compulsive eating that can lead to unnecessary overweight and obesity.

Our tendency has too often been to blame dieters rather than face the failure of our methods. We must consider that our continued belief in dieting as the solution for unwanted and unhealthy fatness is causing much more harm than good, increasing health risks, and triggering eating habits that actually encourage the weight gain that we fear.

In the past ten years the popular press has finally begun to leak this conclusion to the general public: weight-loss diets are doomed to fail. By now most people are aware of the discouraging statistics: 95 percent of all weight lost through dieting is regained, usually with added pounds. Furthermore, yo-yo dieting (losing, regaining, losing, regaining) not only contributes to a gradual increase in weight gain over time, but to greater health risks in general. Even obese persons who might benefit from a lower weight suffer more strain when pounds lost through dieting are regained than if they had not been lost in the first place.

That dieting is a no-win effort is no longer a debatable topic in the scientific community. In the early 1990s, the National Institute of Health clearly reported that there is no such thing as a successful weight-loss diet. "It is easy to take weight off obese people with a low-calorie diet, but nearly 100 percent eventually regain their excess weight," said Dr. John Brunzell, winner of the NIH Award for Excellence in Clinical Research. Despite this, reducing diets continue to be embraced by the lay public and prescribed by physicians. Why is this?

WHY DO PEOPLE CONTINUE TO DIET?

In part 1, I mentioned some of the reasons why dieting still flourishes when it is so clearly not a good idea. For one thing, we know very well that the diet industry's powerful campaigns are very persuasive both in encouraging weight dissatisfaction and in urging us to believe diets can work. Even physicians are not immune to the kind of mass marketing that fuels weightist attitudes across our culture. But for physicians, there are additional pressures. Many patients desperately press their doctors for behavioral and pharmaceutical help in achieving weight loss. In addition, a physician's concern about the rise in medical problems associated with excess weight is usually genuine and appropriate. Frustrated and unable to view the problem as one that can be solved, many of our nation's medical leaders persist in prescribing diets.

I find most physicians feel as baffled and helpless about weight issues as any layperson. Having spent twenty-five years practicing in this arena, I understand their frustration in that weight so often defies our determination to control it. But there is no excuse for continuing to recommend an approach that has consistently been proven to fail. Doing so tragically reinforces a very damaging message—that 95 percent of all dieters must be doing something wrong—rather than acknowledging that dieting itself, as a weight-loss method, is intrinsically flawed.

From both a scientific and philosophical perspective, shifting the focus to prescriptions for healthy lifestyle choices, thereby eliminating the focus on dieting and weight loss, is the only realistic public-health policy available today. Yet many physicians have trouble making this shift, even though the end result will be a far healthier population. Dietitian Ellyn Satter said it simply: "We cannot get people to lose weight, and we should not promise them that we will try. We can help people learn to eat. We can help them discover enjoyment in moving their bodies. And we can help them let their weight find its own level in response to this."

Doctors want to help patients fulfill their wishes whenever possible. It takes courage to tell patients that weight loss is not something you can promise them—but that if they will learn to eat well and develop their fitness level, their body will settle at a weight that is normal and healthy for them. This is not what the American public wants to be told, but it is the most honest and respectful advice we can offer to anyone, at any size.

SHOULD TRULY FAT CHILDREN BE PUT ON DIETS?

It is possible that as new medications (without damaging side effects) are developed, treatment that intervenes in the workings of the internal weight regulatory system may become a medical option. Such medications would be similar to the antidepressant medications that have dramatically changed the face of mental-health treatment. In the meantime, dieting is no better as a treatment for obesity than for the twenty pounds Aunt Sue put on last winter or the five pounds your child may want to lose before starting junior high school.

A HEALTHIER EQUATION

When people hear or read about genetic predisposition for body size and that dieting is not recommended, they worry that this endorses a "don't worry, be flabby" approach to life. Nothing could be further from the truth. As a mom, I am as concerned about the health, strength, fitness, well-being, and longevity of my children, their father, and myself as you are with your family. Rather than leaving us without options, knowing that kids come in all sizes and accepting that dieting does not have a good outcome open the door to embracing the important, realistic options.

The negative results of dieting are so predictable that I often tell teenagers that if they want to have weight problems as adults, the best means is to become dieters now. Our job as parents is to teach our kids what to do instead. Guidance for eating well and developing a lifestyle that promotes fitness are the topics of the following two chapters. But as kids are faced daily with advertisements, magazine articles, and books promoting the latest, greatest weight-loss scheme, they need first to understand inside and out exactly why dieting is not a good idea. Read on to learn an effective method for passing along this message.

TEACHABLE MOMENTS

Once you look for them, you will be amazed at how frequently opportunities arise to teach your child that dieting is not a good idea. I guarantee there will be innumerable occasions when you will encounter outrageous diet advertisements on TV, in magazines, on billboards, in the newspaper, and on the radio. While in the grocery checkout line, consider counting the magazine covers that offer promising weight-loss tips inside. Any of these encounters can cue a conversation about dieting. Let your child know that with all of the messages promoting dieting, you want to teach her the truth about it.

TALKING WITH KIDS

Tell your child that to understand why dieting is not a good idea, we have to remember that hunger is one of the five drives that keeps us alive. In order to live we must satisfy five basic needs. See if your child can name these: *sleep, water, oxygen, food, and warmth (shelter)*. We are so dependent on these, we cannot stop ourselves from trying to fulfill our need for them— at least not for long. In fact, if basic needs are not fully satisfied, even for a short time, we can expect to see very predictable negative consequences. The following activity will allow your child to consider sleep deprivation, dehydration, and experience an "air diet," learning first hand why restricting food intake is not an effective means to achieve lasting weight loss.

BODY LIFT

Consider sleep deprivation

Ask your child to think about how many hours of sleep she needs per night to be well rested. Then ask her what would happen if one night she lost three of those hours of sleep. Most kids know they would be sleepy the next day, not quite as alert, and maybe irritable.

Next ask her what would happen if she lost three hours of

sleep every night for a whole week (with no naps)—or for a whole month. Kids know there would be predictable consequences. After a week or more of lost sleep, she would be tired all the time, even after just waking in the morning, craving sleep all day, and looking for a chance to take a nap. Concentration would be difficult, and she would be crabby and uncomfortable—maybe even sick. After a month of sleep deficit, this response would be severe. If your child has ever had too little sleep (whose child has not?), she has already learned from experience what happens when sleep needs aren't met.

Now ask her what would happen when, after all this time, she could finally sleep all she wanted. Would she be immediately content with her normal sleep schedule? Most kids will know instinctively that they would want to sleep extra hours, probably for many nights in a row. In fact, it might take two to three weeks to get back on track. Teenagers demonstrate this every weekend, and we say they are "catching up" after a week of early wake-ups for school. When sleep needs aren't met, we try to make up for the hours we missed when we finally have the chance.

Consider dehydration

Now ask your child how she would feel if she was told that for a whole day she could have only eight tablespoons of water (half a cup) every four hours from morning to night. It is likely that, even without ever having experienced this, she will know instinctively that she would be thinking a lot about liquids and feeling very thirsty all day that day. Ask her to imagine having to take an important test that day, and find out if she thinks she would have any trouble concentrating. She will understand this kind of limitation would be frustrating! Even so, you can tell her that one day without water would not result in true dehydration. Nonetheless, when an external restriction is put on something so vital as water, we automatically crave what is missing. Now ask your child what she would do when there were no more restrictions on liquids at bedtime. She will know she would want to guzzle *extra* water.

The Air Diet

Ask your child if she thinks a similar result would occur if she didn't get enough air to breathe. Suggest that she try a little "air diet" that you have learned about. In a gentle, teasing way, tell her you've noticed her cheeks have looked especially rosy lately. Then ask if she has heard the latest style is to have kind of blue or grayish skin tone. Since oxygen is what gives cheeks that rosy glow, tell her she would surely be better off if she'd cut back on her breathing so her face coloring could be more blue. Of course, she will need some air to live, but surely she could cut back. It will be worth it to have the "right look."

If you have a drinking straw, tell your child to plug her nose and breathe entirely through a straw. If you lack a straw, you can accomplish the same end by having your child plug one side of her nose, close her mouth, and breathe entirely through one nostril. Laughing is cheating! While she is on her air diet, you can fill the time with anything that requires no talking and a little concentration. This could be nonsense, like writing the names of family members backwards, or academic, like doing a few math problems. For enhanced effect, this could be some form of mild physical exercise that will increase her need for oxygen and exaggerate the effects of air deprivation. Continue the air diet (no longer than a few minutes) until you see that she is experiencing the same expected, predictable consequences she noted with sleep deprivation and fluid restriction: preoccupation with breathing, craving air, difficulty concentrating on anything else, crabbiness, etc. If she "goes off" her air diet before it's time, be sure to tease her, saying, "Wait a minute! Don't you want to have the 'right look'? Where is your willpower?"

When you begin to notice signs of discomfort from restricted breathing, it is time to tell her she can go off her air diet. While she is taking big gulps of air, be sure to comment that it is expected that she will breathe extra hard when oxygen has been deprived.

As your child is still catching her breath, you can review what has been learned. When any of the five basic needs are deprived, we can always expect

- A powerful craving to satisfy the need
- Difficulty concentrating on anything except what is missing
- Discomfort—the whole thing makes us crabby or irritable
- Wanting more than a normal amount to make up for what was missing, once we finally get to have as much as we want

Restricted Hunger

Your child may not know it yet, but she has already learned the reasons why restricting hunger for weight loss is doomed. Paraphrase the following information to make the connection perfectly clear:

We hear a lot of messages these days telling us we should lose weight by going on a diet. Dieting has become very common, even among people who are already slim. With all of the pressure to join in, it's important to ask whether restricting hunger to "diet" is a good idea. Does it work?

Since hunger is one of the five basic drives that keep us alive, it's logical that restricting our hunger causes more problems than it solves. That is what happened for the Namuh when they went on diets: "They became so hungry! When they finally let themselves eat, planning, of course, to eat just a little, they couldn't stop—not for a long time and not until well after they were quite stuffed."

Dieting for weight loss does cause big problems. It is not a good idea. Here are things you should tell your child to expect if she restricts her hunger:

1. A dieter is almost constantly thinking about food. Being on a diet makes it hard to concentrate or think about anything else.
2. There is a huge craving for food, especially fast energy foods like sweets and high-fat foods.
3. Unmet hunger is very uncomfortable. Dieters have little patience, are crabby, and may be self-centered.
4. A huge hunger occurs when dieters go off their diet plan. They will often gobble food very fast and feel they cannot get enough. It is normal to eat an extra large amount of food when going off a diet. Dieters may not know they are full until they are stuffed!
5. The longer a diet lasts and the more times a person diets, the more overeating or "stuffing" occurs after the diet. The most common cause of overeating is dieting.
6. After losing weight on a diet, most people regain the weight, plus added pounds.
7. The more people diet, the harder it is to tell when they are full and when they are still hungry. They may always feel hungry, even if they are not. If they stop dieting long enough, they may get back their normal hunger sensor, but some people never do.

Many diets work at first. People lose weight for a time, but after a while they can expect to overeat to make up for it.

What should I tell my child when her aunt Sue is dieting?

Given the continued prevalence of dieting, it is extremely likely your child will know someone—maybe even you—who diets. This often comes up in school settings, when students learn the lessons in my *Healthy Body Image* curriculum and then watch teachers in the lunchroom eating only carrot sticks and talking about their latest diets. As usual with kids, the best response is an honest one. Tell them that until recently, it was not well known that dieting is not a good idea. This means there are still a lot of people who have not learned about it. In short, you can handle it in the same way that you might handle your child's question about why Grandpa smokes or why Aunt Jane still spends hours in the sun to get a tan.

What should I tell my child about diet advertisements?

It is hard to go through a single day without seeing or hearing an advertisement for weight-loss products or programs. Once your child has learned why eating according to a weight-loss plan doesn't work, she will need help to understand why these advertisements are still allowed to exist. You can tell her that Congress is passing new laws to strictly regulate advertisements for weight-loss programs, modeled after laws that now regulate cigarette ads. Until these take effect, you can help your child resist the seductive, but false and misleading messages they present. Be sure to do the activities in lesson 9 on media literacy, one of which is specifically designed to strengthen your child's immunity to diet ads.

BODY-ESTEEM AFFIRMATIONS

When your child has learned the essential message of this lesson, she will relate to affirmations like these:

- Dieting in hopes of losing weight is not a good idea. You may lose weight at first, but after a while you will overeat to make up for it.
- The best way to avoid overeating is to choose wholesome food and avoid undereating.
- If I'm still hungry, I haven't eaten enough.

Lesson 7:
Eating Well for Healthy Weight

With reasonable care, our children's bodies will grow and maintain a weight that is right for each of them. But what is reasonable care? Wholesome eating and physical fitness are needed to make this equation work. Eating well, a pleasure for most people, means eating and enjoying a variety of foods that taste good, provide energy, and satisfy nutritional needs. It also means tuning in to ourselves to know what we want to eat, when we are hungry, and when we have had enough. Eating well is neither anxiety provoking or conflict laden. It requires some thoughtfulness and attention, but is a part of life that can flow easily and naturally for those who have access to a variety of wholesome food and a basic respect for nutrition. At the same time, eating well can be unbelievably difficult for those who either lack good food, care little about balanced nutrition, or have become anxious in their relationship to food.

Many Americans do not eat well. The results include inadequate nutrition that may affect health, and/or eating compulsions that make people feel afraid, angry, or otherwise out of control around food. Sometimes the result can be extreme, leading to eating disorders and unhealthy fatness. The goal of this lesson is to help your kids feel good about eating well, to know how to make healthy choices, to carry out that intention, and to maintain responsibility for their own hunger despite contrary pressures around them. Ideally, this could be expressed as, "I am the best authority on what I want to eat, on when I'm hungry, and on when I'm full. I make a reasonable effort to eat a variety of healthy foods to satisfy my hunger." Eating well maintains body esteem in its purest form.

GROWN-UPS, KIDS, AND EATING

When feeding kids, it works best to know who is responsible for what. Ellyn Satter, a noted authority in childhood nutrition and feeding, is known for clarifying responsibilities when it comes to kids and eating. Her books, particularly *Secrets of Feeding a Healthy Family*, should be required reading for parents in prenatal classes. (For a list of Satter's books, see appendix D.)

Satter says the division of labor that works best is

- Parents are responsible for what, when, and where a child is fed.
- Children are responsible for deciding how much to eat and whether or not to eat a particular food.

This respectful, commonsense approach is based on the belief that parents need to do what children cannot: (1) choose and provide nutritious, varied foods, (2) structure regular, predictable, and pleasant eating times, and (3) model what it means to have a positive, "grown-up" relationship with food. It is also based on the belief that children must do what parents cannot: maintain the integrity of their own experience. Your child alone knows what tastes good or bad to her, and how much she needs to eat to satisfy her hunger. Positive body esteem requires maintenance of the ability to listen to internal cues, rather than external messages. Trust your child, and she will learn to trust herself.

This means that your child will not be able to do her job unless you do yours: provide a wholesome selection of food at predictable times, in an appealing manner, on a routine basis.

Until the age of twelve or thirteen, your child is almost completely reliant on you and other adults in her life to obtain and offer a selection of fresh and prepared food that is healthy and appealing. While teens develop more independence, their feeding needs do not really change. Throughout their years at home, kids do best when grown-ups take the lead in providing wholesome food and expecting kids to eat regular, healthy meals. As adults, we need to be prepared to make choices about the nutritional contribution of the foods we provide.

THE TRUTH ABOUT JUNK FOOD

*"Junk" food is everywhere. When I see the signs,
I always think, "Let's stop and get some!"*
—second-grade student

Junk food is a common term for food that is low in nutrient value when we consider how many calories it contains. Junk food is an unfortunate label, because it suggests that these foods are bad for us and that we are bad to eat them. But the problem with these foods is not that they are toxic in any way. They are not even worthless, since they generally provide calories, which we need for energy. Some people live a long life eating little else. Even so, few people doubt the benefits of more healthful eating. So the big problem with junk food is, because it tastes so good, is dirt cheap, and is available at every turn, it too often ends up taking the place of more nutritious foods that are needed by our bodies.

Here are some trivia questions to test your knowledge of junk food.

• White Castle was the first fast-food restaurant. McDonald's was the second. When did the first McDonald's restaurant open? (The first McDonald's restaurant opened in 1957 in Iowa.)

• How many fast-food restaurants are there in the world today? (Counting only the big three, McDonald's, KFC, and Pizza Hut, there are 52,786 as of 2003.)

• How many kinds of potato chips could you buy forty-five years ago? (One—available in a small section at the grocery store. Today? Hundreds.)

• What is the number one selling item today in American grocery stores? (Soda. One can contains about a quarter cup sugar and about 170 empty calories.)

• Packaged, ready-to-eat junk food as we know it today did not exist only forty years ago.

The way people eat has changed since the *mass marketing* of ready-to-eat foods. Sweets and tasty high-fat foods have always been enjoyed. But until recently, they were almost entirely homemade. Treats have only been packaged and sold ready-to-eat at a low cost for a few years. In much the same way that advertising has influenced our attitudes about looks, the clever advertising of junk food has influenced attitudes about what we eat.

TEACHING KIDS TO EAT WELL

Make eating well a priority

It may seem like this lesson requires too much time and trouble to put into practice. As a working parent of kids who are involved in constant extracurricular activities (many of which seem to conflict with mealtimes), a nonstop social calendar, and the occasional homework, I am completely sympathetic. But the reward for making eating well a priority is a child who has learned the essential equation for a lifetime of confidence that she is well nourished and that her weight is right for her. This is no small accomplishment in today's world. The amount of mental anguish, diminished self-esteem, and ill health that results from eating problems and body angst takes far more time and energy than learning the business of competent eating from the start. Consider the effort you put into helping your child eat well as an investment in her lifelong well-being. As a bonus for parents who have struggled with their own body image and eating concerns, learning to confidently provide healthy meals and model healthy eating may be a gift to yourself as well.

Parents who lack financial resources face additional feeding challenges. But I work with children from elite private schools to low-income neighborhoods, and I find it is less often a lack of money and more often a lack of time, energy, and education about positive eating habits that gets in the way. Regardless of income, think about whether you carry out your role as food supplier in a way that encourages or impedes the goal of healthy eating. If you decide you need some remedial help, don't feel bad. It's a tough world in which to be a healthy eater. The effort is worth it.

Plan for times to eat, and times not to eat

Kids (and grown-ups too, for that matter) need regular, predictable times to eat, followed by times to do things other than eat. Essentially this boils down to eating at mealtime, rather than taking a grazing approach to feeding. Grazing is not inherently bad, but most experts agree that it is problematic for most people. Unfortunately, with such busy schedules, grazing has become the default eating style for many Americans. Grabbing food on the run seems normal. This means that for a significant number of our kids, the notion of a structured time to feed themselves, with attention paid to wholesome food, seems novel, if not downright peculiar. Since eating is a tradition passed from one generation to the next, it behooves us to think about how what we are instilling in our children will affect our grandchildren.

The fact is that in order to satisfy hunger with a good variety of nutritious foods in amounts that are beneficial for growth, some kind of feeding structure is essential for kids and adults. It becomes very hard to know whether nutrition needs are being met when feeding is ongoing throughout the day or occurs on demand. Even healthy snacks and beverages that are eaten "whenever" spoil hunger for meals and keep kids from working up enough of an appetite to be interested in the varied nutritious foods that are offered at breakfast, lunch, and dinner. In addition, there is a confusing psychological aspect to grazing. By the end of the day, we may feel either that we never really ate, even though we may have consumed a large number of calories, or that we ate all day, even if we ate neither enough calories nor a good balance of foods.

Many adult men and women who feel out of control with food have never learned or have lost sight of the need for some kind of structure for eating. Part of learning to eat competently includes knowing it is worthwhile to save our appetites in anticipation of an enjoyable meal. Kids who are not sure when that next meal will be are often excessively preoccupied with food, begging for snacks to curb the smallest amount of hunger, not willing to trust that food will be available for a larger appetite. Other kids who are uncertain about when or what they will be fed may learn to feel in control by tuning out hunger cues, developing a worrisome disinterest in food even when it is provided. Confusion and anxiety about when and where the next meal will be and what will be eaten increases without a predictable plan.

The length of the interval between eating times will depend somewhat on your child's age. Most growing children need a shot of energy about every two and a half to three hours. While this should never be rigid, it usually boils down to three reliable meals and two to three snacks planned in such a way that they do not spoil hunger for meals. As kids get older, they may comfortably go three to five hours without food, and snacks may or may not be as vital. If, however, intervals between meals are as long as five to six hours or longer, close attention should be paid to the hunger that will build, as this is a setup for eating that feels uncontrolled. Countless adults and teens who come home from work or school too hungry to wait for a meal to be prepared suffer from such a scenario.

It is too much to expect that hunger that has been held back too long should be held even longer once food is in sight. Unfortunately, quick relief often comes in the form of ready-to-eat treats that kill appetite without supplying nutrients. The worst outcome is for those who do not recognize that the problem is not lack of willpower, but the natural outcome of hunger that has been put on hold for too long. Far better for parents and kids to learn to respect their hunger cycles, and plan snacks or mealtimes accordingly.

Reasonable intervals between eating are extremely important in teaching children self-confidence, trust, discipline and self-management. From the time that our infants demonstrate they can handle a (flexible) schedule for feeding, our job is to reinforce their security in learning that they do not need to be munching tidbits or thinking about their next snack all the time in order to be well fed. They can feel free to go off and play or work, engaging deeply in other activities, confident that feeding will happen. Having distinct times to eat and times to do other things when we are not eating hugely reinforces the value of both. It sends a message that says, "Nourishing your body matters and deserves its own designated time," while at the same time saying, "There are things for you to do in the world that do not include eating. These also matter and deserve your undivided attention as well." This is an aspect of maturation that is unfortunately lost on many adults today. As food has been packaged for increased portability, we routinely eat whatever, whenever. Children benefit from having adults in their lives who model a healthy, balanced relationship with food, including times to eat it and times for the rest of our lives.

Having designated times to eat meals or snacks together is a communal activity that strengthens family ties, improves relationships, promotes communication, and lets kids know you are invested in them. If you have allowed family mealtimes to lapse, then consider this: Teens who report they have regular family meals do better in school, have better relationships with peers, are less depressed, and are less likely to use drugs. As a working parent, I know that the list of things that can interfere with family meals (which can mean any two or more people eating together, preferably including an adult) is endless (including events that schools schedule over the dinner hour!). I am very familiar with the challenge of treats that are passed out to kids by other kids and other adults with no regard for spoiling appetites needed for the next mealtime. Still, it is up to you to make meals, especially family meals, a priority.

To eat or not to eat is not the question

You do not have to worry if your child will want to eat. She will. If kids are not eating, if they are losing weight or appear disinterested in eating for more than a few days, this is a sign that something is wrong, and you should seek professional assessment. It is the job of children to *grow*, and even fat children should not be dropping pounds unless you are absolutely sure they are getting all the nutrients they need, are not denying their hunger, and are not exercising compulsively. Keep in mind that different children have different appetites, ranging from very small to very large. Fluctuations in appetite from day to day and week to week are not cause for concern. Beyond this, not wanting to eat may reflect a medical problem or a mental-health concern, such as depression or anxiety (both of which can interfere with hunger). Some kids have a need to express something that is difficult for them, and the only way they can find to do it is by not eating. If we try to force them to eat more or less than they are hungry for, this will cause problems, not relieve them. If your child fails to eat enough to fulfill her nutritional needs and is not growing normally, you should seek help to find out why.

Does it really matter what kids eat, as long as they have energy?

In a world in which we are surrounded at every turn by low-nutrient, high-energy treats, feeding children well can be a challenge.

One summer day when my kids were in elementary school, they were fantasizing what it would be like to have nothing but treats to choose from, from morning to night, with no limitations. My children were not strangers to treats, but knew them primarily as fillers—something to fill that little bubble of space that might remain after most of their hunger had been spent on higher-nutrient foods. I decided, just for fun, to let them try out their fantasy. They had a great time planning what they might want to eat, and we made a trip to the store the night before to be sure we had what they wanted on hand. Their choices all fell into the categories of rich, sugary desserts and fried salty snacks— typical junk-food fare: candy, cookies, chips, and soda.

When their day began, the kids woke with excitement and quickly began to indulge. All was going as planned until about four in the afternoon when my daughter somewhat sheepishly asked if we could have some "real" food for dinner. Even today my daughter remembers her surprise at realizing she had had her fill of treats and that what she hungered for was something of greater substance. I'd like to say this is how I planned it, but I

Because of their intense stimulating flavor, low cost, ready availability, and promotion through mass marketing, low-nutrient, high-fat/high-sugar foods fit today's casual, on-the-go lifestyles. Even so, an overabundance of these foods interferes with balanced eating, as their selection crowds out hunger needed for high-nutrient foods.

was as surprised as she that her body had so quickly and loudly exerted its wisdom. If you decide to try this experiment, I can't guarantee your child will learn the same lesson in so short a time. But anytime your child is happily, completely stuffed with treats is a very good time to consider the following questions: *"Would this be a good way to eat all the time? Why not?"*

The first response you are likely to hear from kids is, "It would make you too fat!" Indeed, this kind of eating does play a part in the unhealthy fatness of some people. However, if you remember lessons 3 and 4, you know this depends on the person and their metabolism. If your children offer this response, it is a great opportunity to review: *Some people live on a diet that is primarily made up of treats and stay thin forever. Other people who are quite fat may eat very few treats.* So there is a more important reason: *You would not get enough of what your body needs for good nutrition.*

This answer will probably seem very boring to your child. The effect of good or poor nutrition is too abstract, and kids are not interested in it. Fortunately they don't need to be, because they have you to choose and provide nutritious food for them at this time of their life. Along the way, they will learn about nutrition and its value, if you make a point to teach them—in part through your commentary, but especially by your example. When they reach the age of choosing for themselves, your efforts will have helped them to become competent, healthy eaters who naturally look for a balanced variety of nutritious foods at regularly scheduled times.

WHAT IS GOOD NUTRITION?

Just about everyone knows that the best way to eat nutritiously is to eat a variety of foods from all the different food groups. The Food Guide Pyramid (see page 171) is the nutrition guide recommended by the U.S. Departments of Agriculture and Health and Human Services. Last revised in 2000, the Food Guide Pyramid recommends the minimum number of servings needed from each of five food groups in order to satisfy our health needs. The pyramid shape shows the relative proportion that each food group should contribute to our total daily food intake. Foods made from grains are considered the foundation, with fruits and vegetables filling in next, followed by foods high in calcium and protein. The top of the pyramid includes what most of us think of as "treats"—foods high in energy, but generally low in nutrient value. The Food Guide Pyramid contains sound advice for all of us to build on.

Every five years these guidelines are revised, which means that as of this writing, committee members are considering changes based on the latest research. By the time you are reading this, the 2005 guidelines may be available. While the overall form of the Food Guide Pyramid will remain, it is likely there will be a few changes based not only on new findings in dietary science but on observations about how the public interprets the current pyramid. Do look for the 2005 revised Food Guide Pyramid, but meanwhile I feel confident in predicting some of the most likely changes:

- The base of the pyramid will strongly emphasize *whole-grain* foods, versus those made with refined white flour and rice. During the milling of refined grains, the healthy bran and germ are removed, leaving a carbohydrate food that is high in energy, but low in nutients. Because these refined grains are lower both in fiber *and* in nutrient density, they are digested quickly and we tend to crave more of them to satisfy hunger. These empty calories have probably contributed to unhealthy weight gain in the American population.

- Fruits and vegetables will be recommended in abundance or in unlimited amounts.

- Rather than lumping all fats together at the top of the pyramid, vegetable, nut, and seed oils will be encouraged, while saturated fats from animal products and trans fats, such as those found in stick margarine and many processed foods, will be strongly discouraged.

- Low-fat dairy products will be recommended more clearly.

- More nuts and seeds will be encouraged as protein foods, along with legumes, fish, and poultry. A suggestion will be made to limit red meats, which are higher in saturated fats.
- Daily exercise will be included as part of the pyramid.

Keeping in mind these new recommendations, you and your child will get what you need if you follow a flexible version of the Food Guide Pyramid. Focus on eating at least the minimum number of servings suggested for each food group. Keep in mind that minimum means *minimum*. This is the lowest number of servings needed to provide the essential vitamins, minerals, fiber, protein, carbohydrates, and fats that your body needs to be healthy. The minimum certainly does not reflect the number of calories you or your child needs to have good energy, maintain a healthy weight, and satisfy hunger and appetite. Most people will need to eat much more than the minimum to adequately fulfill these needs most of the time. How much more will depend on each person's internal cues at any given time on any given day, based on trusting our body's integrity and internal hunger regulation. If you try to eat less than your hunger and appetite dictate, you will trigger the internal food-deprivation mechanisms. The idea is to eat enough. Eating enough is completely natural. But in today's world it requires tuning out external messages in order to tune in to inner signals.

One problem with the Food Guide Pyramid is that it advises a limited range of servings. Even though the upper limit suggested is very generous and probably reflects far more food than 90 percent of the population would ever want to eat in a day, the existence of an upper limit sends the message that we cannot completely trust our internal hunger regulators to tell us when we are full. Rather than encouraging us to tune in to ourselves, to pay attention to the taste and feel of food in our mouth and stomach, to be aware of internal signals that tell us we want more or have eaten enough, an upper limit warns us that we may not be trustworthy. It wrongly suggests that we need an external guide to define "too much." This is problematic, because *any* external restriction on basic drives encourages anxiety, preoccupation, and craving for more of whatever is limited—even if the amount allowed is generous.

Still, people worry about this. They ask, "If adults and kids have lost touch with internal hunger cues through a history of unhealthy eating, don't they need to be told how much is too much?" This question reflects a double bind. It is not possible for people to reconnect with internal hunger cues if external rules are imposed, causing them to feel they cannot trust themselves. In treating children or adults who have lost touch with their ability to know when they are full, it is both a huge relief and very scary for them when I recommend that we eliminate the rules defining too much food. Most are sure that they will eat the entire house and more without these rules. In reality, many do eat excessive amounts for a short while—stocking up as their psyches wait nervously for the next restrictive diet to be imposed. But if such individuals can maintain their courage and continue to fill up with a reasonable selection of wholesome foods, eventually their subconscious minds register what is happening: *they are free to eat according to their own internal hunger.* At this point, something almost magical happens (or so it seems to those who have come to see themselves as insatiable). Suddenly, because they no longer need to eat in anticipation of the time when they will be cut off, they no longer need to eat it all right now. They begin to notice when they are full. They begin to trust that they can save some for later or can share their food, knowing they can get more if they choose. When offered nutritious food and an opportunity to self-regulate, less is enough. Body esteem is restored.

By now you have noticed my frequent use of the phrase *reasonable care* regarding feeding your children. I have also recommended a balanced variety of wholesome foods, using the Food Guide Pyramid as a guide. But how does this translate into everyday life? If you already have a way that works to cover the bases for your family's nutritional needs, then you are ahead of the game. For anyone whose efforts are not working, here are some recommendations.

1. Offer multiple servings of foods that are made primarily from grain (preferably whole grain) at each meal. For example, at breakfast you might have whole-grain cereal, rice, bread, waffles, pancakes, or muffins. Lunch and dinner might include any of these as well, but also pasta or other whole-grain noodles, rice, grits, tortillas, popcorn, and whole-grain crackers. In addition, grain foods can be offered as planned snacks after school or before bed. If kids eat only one serving of grain at each of their three meals, plus as two snacks, they will already have five servings. Since grain foods are generally popular, it is common for kids to want to eat two to three servings at a sitting, which means they should easily be able to eat more than the minimum. There is absolutely no need for you to keep track of how much whole grain your child is eating as long as he is eating grain at most meals and snacks most of the time. There should be no limit on the number of servings offered, *as long as she is eating a wide enough variety of foods to satisfy nutritional needs from other food groups.*

  Without a doubt, the closer grains are to the plant, the better. Kids who are provided with whole-grain breads, pasta, cereal, and rice from an early age grow up happily eating these foods as teens. If kids have gotten used to white-flour pasta, white rice, and white bread, they may need to develop their appetite for these more wholesome options gradually. Be flexible, but firm and persistent in helping kids visualize that refined grains are relatively *empty of nutrients,* while rougher, browner whole-grain foods are rich with goodness their bodies need.

2. In addition to grain, offer one or two vegetables, a fruit, some protein (meat, nut butters, eggs, tofu, cheese, or legumes), a calcium food (low-fat milk, yogurt, cheese), and some vegetable or seed-based fat at each meal. Butter or oil can be added for flavor or used in the cooking process. Fats are also available in cheese, many meats, peanut butter, olives, and avocados, as well as treats, such as cookies or chips. If you don't want to eat protein or vegetables at breakfast, just double up at other meals or snacks. For most, making it a goal to eat five per day of fruits and vegetables will be the single most important thing you can do to improve your nutrition and chances for a healthy weight. If you are unsure what foods belong to each group, get a basic book on nutrition at the library or find this information online.

3. Give children independence and control through offering food choices. However, when offering choices, make them nutritionally comparable. For example, if your main purpose is entertainment, cake or french fries are pretty equal. If it's time for lunch, either a turkey sandwich or spinach lasagna offer good nutrition. On the other hand, for dinner, a choice between a veggie stir-fry, pineapple, and milk, or nachos and a Coke is not comparable.

4. After you and your kids have eaten a balance of foods that meet nutritional requirements, then eat more from any of

the five food groups at any meal until your hunger and energy needs are satisfied.

5. If dessert is desired, eat it after hunger has been nearly satiated.

6. If you or your kids have room for lots of treats after a meal (more than a couple cookies or a scoop of ice cream), you may not have yet eaten enough of the main menu. Suggest more lunch or dinner rather than more treats. In practice, I teach children to think of hunger like money; that is, for most of us, there is a finite amount of both. While we enjoy spending some money on short-term gratification, entertainment, and trinkets, we know that if we spend too much this way, there may not be enough remaining for items of substance that have more lasting value. In the same way, treats are a delightful part of life, but since hunger is limited, for good health the biggest portion of it needs to be spent on foods that have high nutrient value.

Children can understand that this approach is not about deprivation, or "good foods / bad foods," but about a mindful use of resources for different purposes. Viewing hunger as a resource is like teaching a child that to save for a bike, she will probably have to limit how many smaller toys she buys. To be a good athlete, student, musician, or physically fit she will need to make decisions about her allocation of free time. Use of time and money are competencies children are accustomed to learning and parents are accustomed to teaching. I often tell kids they might want to save a "little bubble" of hunger for a low-nutrient treat. If they find that they have hunger left over for more than a couple cookies or a dessert, they probably left more than a little bubble. In this case, they might want to spend remaining hunger on the more nutrient dense foods from the meal.

Another question that helps kids tune in to themselves is, "Are you hungry, or do you feel like entertaining yourself with food?" Most of us enjoy entertaining ourselves with food. The point is to be aware that this is what we are doing and to maintain a balance, just as we do with any division of responsibility versus play.

7. You will be well ahead of the game if you think of snacks as small meals and choose foods that get most of their food value from one of the five food groups—peanut butter on a whole-grain bagel, cereal and fruit, veggies and dip. Again, spend most of your hunger on wholesome food before munching on high-energy, low-nutrient foods. At the same time, there's no reason for kids to avoid treats that primarily supply only calories and few nutrients *if they generally eat well.*

8. Never turn guidelines like these into rigid rules. If eating-disorder, body-image, and weight-concern specialists have learned anything in the past fifteen years, it is that rigid rules that aim to control eating are the cause of most types of disordered eating. Rules tend to make us feel we have been "good" or "bad," and are usually accompanied by shame, guilt, and the inclination to rebel. Guidelines are more about what works and what doesn't work over time to achieve balanced eating. If you move in the direction of following these guidelines closely but not rigidly, it is extremely likely that your children will grow into adults who enjoy eating well, without unnecessary anxiety or undue attention. This means that if one day you and your kids blow all your hunger for dinner on banana splits because you stayed too long at the beach, everyone was starving, and the only available food was at the ice-cream stand, then you can enjoy it without worry, knowing most dinners you eat include all the basics. At the same time, if for whatever rea-

son, you routinely miss out on wholesome eating at predictable mealtimes, then it's going to be hard for your kids to learn what wholesome eating is—and that it is an important value in their lives and yours.

9. Remember to think positively. This is a basic principle of life. Even when your wish is to "stop eating so much chocolate," or "stop eating compulsively," or "stop dieting," this will not occur until you decide to start making a positive, contrasting choice. For example, "start eating the minimum daily nutritional requirements," or "start satisfying hunger completely at distinct, regular meals."

In an ideal world children do not need this instruction to ensure their health. Given a variety of hearty foods and a wholesome environment, children have proven they will naturally eat when they are hungry and stop when they are full, choosing foods that provide balanced nutrition without conflict or anxiety. Unfortunately, this is not the environment in which most of today's children develop. Instead, kids must learn from an early age to navigate in a sea of cheap, ready to eat, taste-stimulating foods packaged and promoted specifically to lure them into over-valuing and craving it. At the same time children hear a never-ending stream of messages about the size and shape their bodies should be, and how to achieve this through manipulation (restriction) of food and exercise. In light of this contamination, children cannot be expected to maintain body esteem and competency as eaters without extra guidance.

THE FOOD GUIDE PYRAMID
Recommended Daily Guidelines for Healthy Eating

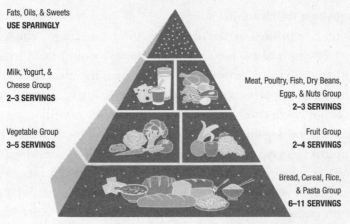

Fats, Oils, & Sweets
USE SPARINGLY

Milk, Yogurt, &
Cheese Group
2–3 SERVINGS

Meat, Poultry, Fish, Dry Beans,
Eggs, & Nuts Group
2–3 SERVINGS

Vegetable Group
3–5 SERVINGS

Fruit Group
2–4 SERVINGS

Bread, Cereal, Rice,
& Pasta Group
6–11 SERVINGS

SOURCE: U.S. Department of Agriculture/U.S. Department of Health and Human Services

BODY LIFT
DO YOU EAT ENOUGH?

You can have your child complete this activity on her own, but it will be more successful if others in the family participate. Photocopy pages 173 and 174 and use them to answer this question: Do you eat enough of what you and your child need to be healthy? The activity can be done in as few as three to four days, but will be more representative of your habits if done for a longer period of time, such as a week.

Each participant will need one photocopy each of page 173 for each day the activity is done to record what is eaten that day. At the end of the recording phase, each of you will graph your results on your copy of page 174. This provides a clear, visual image, showing whether or not you are eating enough from each of the food groups most of the time. You will also quickly see if there are food groups on which you should spend more of your hunger.

Suggestions for this activity

Don't be confused by the meaning of "one serving," which is merely a unit of measurement that increases our flexibility in distributing food over several meals. It does not mean that one serving is the correct amount to have in one sitting. It certainly does not mean that one serving should necessarily fill us up or that several servings suggest overeating. In fact, it would be impossible to eat even the minimum of six or more servings of grain in a day if we did not eat several servings at a time. For example, I routinely eat two or even three servings of whole-grain cereal, fruit, nuts, and milk at one time to satisfy my hunger. This wholesome eating is a great start on the daily nutrients I need. Filling up in this way pays off, giving me the freedom to go about my morning without being distracted by food cravings.

Help your child understand servings in an uncomplicated way. Let kids count one piece of bread, one bowl of cereal, a scoop of rice, a small pile of pasta, one fruit, small piles of veggies, a glass of milk, a piece of chicken, the amount of tuna it takes to cover a piece of bread, etc., as one serving. The last thing you want is for your child to become obsessive about measuring serving sizes. Unless your child eats either very large or particularly small portions, then "some" is a good enough approximation to qualify for a serving. On the other hand, if your child happily eats half of a chicken or, in contrast, one bite, she will need a little direction to understand these as more or less than one serving. This should be offered as information only and without any suggestion of judgment. For example, "If

DO YOU EAT ENOUGH?
DAILY FOOD INTAKE

FOOD GROUP	BREAKFAST	LUNCH	DINNER	SNACKS Morning Afternoon Evening	C O U N T
GRAINS cereals, rice, pasta, bread, tortillas, grits, popcorn					
VEGETABLES corn, peas, beans, beets, potatoes, carrots, broccoli, lettuce, tomatoes, green pepper, avocadoes, mushrooms, sprouts, etc.					
FRUITS apples, bananas, oranges, melons, grapes, pineapple, peaches, pears, berries, etc.					
DAIRY milk products, such as milk, low-fat ice cream, yogurt, etc. (If made with cream and added sugar, count also as fats and sweets.)					
PROTEIN meats, cheese (hard and cottage), eggs, nuts, peanut butter, tofu, soy milk, brown beans, and other legumes					
FATS, OILS, SWEETS butter, margarine, oils, mayonnaise, plus foods combined with fats or sugars so most of their energy comes from these foods					

A full-size printable version is available at www.bodyimagehealth.org

- Mark the number of servings you ate each day from each food group.
- Reach to the gray for the minimum each day!

1. **Do you eat enough from each food group?**   2. **If not, how can you make room for what you need?**

Servings per day of grains, preferably whole grains

Day	1	2	3	4	5	6	7	8	9	10	11	12
1												
2												
3												
4												
5												
6												
7												

Servings per day of vegetables

Day	1	2	3	4	5	6	7	8	9	10	11	12
1												
2												
3												
4												
5												
6												
7												

Servings per day of fruits

Day	1	2	3	4	5	6	7	8	9	10	11	12
1												
2												
3												
4												
5												
6												
7												

Servings per day of protein

Day	1	2	3	4	5	6	7	8	9	10	11	12
1												
2												
3												
4												
5												
6												
7												

Servings per day of dairy

Day	1	2	3	4	5	6	7	8	9	10	11	12
1												
2												
3												
4												
5												
6												
7												

Servings per day of fats and sweets

Day	1	2	3	4	5	6	7	8	9	10	11	12
1												
2												
3												
4												
5												
6												
7												

one serving of chicken is about the size of a deck of cards, then how many servings do you think there are in this much chicken?" or, "If a serving of rice is about the size of my fist, do you think one bite of rice would contain the nutrients of one serving?" The only reason to count servings is to help kids see if they are eating enough from the five food groups.

Your child will sometimes need help to know which foods belong to which group or groups. Besides learning to distinguish vegetables and fruits, combination foods can be tricky even for adults who do not know the ingredients of many foods. Many foods will need to be listed in more than one category. For example, spaghetti with red sauce and meatballs is grain (spaghetti), vegetable (tomato sauce), and meat (meatballs). Ice cream is milk and fat/sugar. Foods that are french fried are listed as fats as well as whatever other category applies.

Have kids record their intake for the previous twenty-four hours at the same time every day. Just before bed is a good time. Both adults and children often forget what they ate, particularly if the day included grazing. Urge your child to stretch her memory in order to be detailed and especially to recall tidbits of candy or raw vegetables, after-school snacks, handheld fruits, or other food eaten on the run.

Plotting the graph and discussing the activity

After food intake has been recorded for several days, count the servings for each food group for each day, and plot these on the graph you have photocopied. Take a look at the sample graphs on pages 239–40 to see what this will look like. (The true story of Cheryl, the woman who completed these graphs, is included in appendix C on pages 235–38.) As you can see, the light gray area indicates the minimum servings of each food group needed to satisfy daily nutrition require-

HEALTHY-EATING CHECKLIST

Eating well means answering "true" to the following:	If any statements are "false," correct problems in these ways:
• Food intake is well balanced across all food groups as a rule. No food groups are consistently neglected.	• Eat additional servings of food from the neglected food groups so that at least the minimum number of servings are eaten from each food group.
• Hunger is satisfied completely. There is no restrictive eating for weight loss.	• Learn about the counterproductive effects of dieting for weight loss. Always satisfy hunger completely with a balanced variety of foods. Trust that through eating well and fitness your body will arrive at a healthy weight for you.
• Hunger is satisfied *primarily* by food chosen from the five main food groups and *not* by several servings chosen from the fats, oils, and sugar group.	• Satisfy hunger completely with foods that are high in nutrition first. This will naturally limit the amount of hunger that remains for treats.
• Energy level is good.	• Make sure that hunger is not restricted for weight loss or because of illness. Those with small appetites who need more energy should choose foods that are more energy dense. Look for foods that contain more nutrients and calories in smaller portions. Nutrient- and energy-rich beverages may be useful supplements.
• There is no sign of depression or anxiety.	• Make sure that hunger is not being restricted for weight loss.
• Weight has been stable over time (or for children, has shown consistent growth).	• Check to make sure other corrections (above) are not needed.
• Overall health is good, and there has been no weight loss that suggests nutritional compromise (females have maintained regular menstrual cycles, etc.).	• Consider other medical or mental-health intervention.

ments. The suggestion states, "Reach to the gray for the minimum each day!" Once you have plotted your results, you can ask the following questions, based on what the graph shows: "Our bodies need the minimum in each food group most days. Am I eating enough?" If so, congratulations! Your body thanks you! If not, why do you think this is? What could you do differently to make sure your body gets what it needs?

I use this activity with people of all ages. It is almost always revealing. I am most surprised by how rare it is to find someone who eats the minimum nutritional requirements—ever, let alone daily! Even people who make a significant effort to eat very well are often below the recommended number of servings in one or two food groups. This is not always a problem, and obviously we can live with less than great nutrition. But adjustments are needed if you or your child cannot answer "true" to any one of the statements in the column on the left in the checklist on page 176. If your response to any of these statements is "false," a corrective response is offered in the column on the right.

BODY-ESTEEM AFFIRMATIONS

When your child understands this essential lesson, she will embrace statements like these:

- My body needs a balanced variety of nutritious food from all the food groups.
- If I spend too much hunger on entertainment foods, I won't have hunger left for the nutritious foods my body needs.
- It's important to save my appetite for food from all the food groups.
- I need to decide for myself when I have eaten enough and when I am full.

- I am wise to the fact that mass marketing can have a strong influence on eating habits. I will remember this when I see great-tasting, but low-nutrient foods advertised.
- I have to make some choices to get enough of the wholesome food my body needs.
- I eat well and am physically fit, so I am confident of my weight.

Lesson 8:
The Fitness Equation

The facts are indisputable: eating well and being fit are the two best things anyone can do for their health at any age. Cardiovascular fitness positively affects every major system in the body, significantly reducing your risk for many major, chronic diseases. Large-muscle fitness means we can stay strong, remain flexible, and maintain stamina well into old age. A proven stress reliever, physical activity improves sleep, increases self-confidence, and reduces depression and anxiety. It burns calories from the food we eat, helping to balance a healthy appetite with a healthy weight. Those with physically active lifestyles report their lives are more interesting and fun than people who are more sedentary, and rate overall quality of life to be significantly higher.

Adults and kids who are physically active report higher self-esteem and less body-image angst than those who are more sedentary. Among adolescent girls, those who are physically active at the highest levels show the highest self-esteem scores. When girls use their physical potential, it empowers them and encourages appreciation for their bodies for reasons other than appearance. Without a doubt, motivation to be strong and fit is one of the most valuable gifts a parent can give to their children.

FITNESS AND THE HEALTHY-WEIGHT EQUATION

Fatness that is a result of a too-sedentary lifestyle poses a health risk that is not taken seriously enough by many American people today. But blaming *fatness* may be misleading since it turns out that fatter people who are *fit* are actually at lower risk for health-related problems than slimmer people who are not fit. Since slimness is not a reasonable goal for everyone, the good news is that *fitness is*. Helping our kids to be healthy means helping them to be fit and strong at any size. This probably goes against the grain of everything you have been taught until now. But as we have learned, when weight loss is set as the goal, for health or any other reason, the long-term success rate is dismal. In the end, far too many Americans today—including children—end up both fat and unfit.

Of course, many fat-bodied kids are not fit—often because of the prejudicial put-downs that are directed at them when they are physically active in public. Our thought until recently has been that if we could just slim these kids down by limiting their eating, they would not be the target of such insults, and their motivation for and participation in physical activity would increase. If only it worked! Given the failure rate of dieting, this approach has only made matters worse, leaving fat children on the sidelines, while weightist attitudes go unchallenged. In stark contrast, when eating well and fitness (at any size) are the goal, then some children will lose weight, some will stay the same, and some will even gain (since muscle weighs more than fat.) The same is true for adults. But *all* children and adults who choose to be strong, fit, and well fed will be healthier, regardless of size, and can be confident the resulting weight is right for them.

The problem is that many of us want the end result to be a slim *look*, versus merely health and vitality. Maybe not fashion-model thin or bodybuilder lean, but slim-*mer* or lean-*er*. This collective notion has become so powerful, people routinely feel that "whatever it takes" to produce the desired result is what we should do. Thus began not only the age of dieting, but also the age of exercising for the purpose of weight loss and bodybuilding. The question is, do we want to encourage our children to invest in this mentality, in which the number one goal is appearance, even if the cost is too often diminished health, an unbalanced lifestyle, insecurity, and loss of well-being? For most parents, this is a no-brainer—in theory. But in reality, if your child is fit and strong but not naturally slim, you may find yourself thinking there is more she should be doing. What if you teach your child to feed herself very well and to be active, strong, and fit, but her healthy weight is not where you have been taught to wish it were or believe it "should" be? This is something that parents need to carefully think about and work through. Otherwise, you may be constantly conflicted about the end goal of fitness for your child.

Physical activity, combined with wholesome eating, is the only equation for determining a person's healthy weight. There is no external standard—not height/weight charts, BMI recommendations, or visual analysis—that can or should be trusted over this formula.

THE FITNESS MOVEMENT

The fitness movement today can seem like just another phase or craze, if you pay attention only to the hype created by commercial advertisers. But at its noncommercial heart, an emphasis on fitness urges a return to natural activity—the kind of movement that allows our body's physiology and chemistry to function properly, as they were engineered to do. A sedentary lifestyle has been possible for large numbers of people only in the last century. It is important that we recognize this and teach our children that inactivity is an abnormal condition for the human body. With today's lifestyle habits, the assumption that children get enough exercise simply by being kids is no longer valid. Many changes in modern society have contributed to a decline in the fitness levels of Americans—more than can be discussed here. But it may help if you are aware of three of these changes.

1. Fitness now requires making a conscious choice for most people.

Archaeologists, anthropologists, and historians have established that our ancestors were very physically active in their everyday lives not only to survive but also for recreation. Times of rest and celebration included cultural games, play, courtship, and religious ceremonies, most of which required varied levels of exertion. By comparison, in our mechanized society, working the large muscles of our bodies to earn a living or to travel from one place to another is no longer part of daily life for most people. But the biggest change has occurred in free-time alternatives. With the introduction of electronic entertainment and sedentary transportation options, we now have to make a conscious choice to be active if we want to prevent free time from eroding our health. This can be very difficult given our busy lives. At the end of our workday, most of us are mentally exhausted and bone tired. We often carry home a lot of small-muscle tension. Collapsing into a captivating, undemanding, sedentary entertainment option can be very appealing. The end result is a huge decline in body movement in the American population.

Sedentary entertainment is so much a part of everyday life for most people, it's hard to recognize that merely limiting the amount of time we allow for it goes a long way toward the solution. The space (and perhaps healthy boredom) that results will almost always lead kids (and adults) to look for something more active to do. In fact, studies on motivating kids to be more active have demonstrated that unplugging them from electronic media options is the most promising method. Parents can and should decide how much time their children (as well as they themselves) will be allowed to plug in to entertainment—and stick to it.

2. The motivation for being active is misguided.

Despite all the health, social, and emotional benefits of physical activity, the number one reason for physical activity given by Americans is to lose weight. For confidence that our weight is healthy, routine physical activity is essential. But if exercise doesn't result in weight loss, disappointment frequently causes people to give it up—along with all its benefits. In the words of one young mother, "I exercised five days a week for three months and didn't lose any weight. I thought, 'What's the point?' "

Holding out weight loss as the carrot for exercising is a mistake that routinely backfires. If people exercise for weight loss but achieve "only" improved health and vitality, they often end up disappointed. "Why bother?" is an all-too-frequent response that sends a lot of people looking for the couch and remote control. Kids who learn to value health, strength, and fitness *in their own right* will be motivated to be active and strong without risking the disappointment that may be tied to a goal weight. More substantial reasons for staying fit can provide a lifetime of freedom and opportunity purchased with strength, stamina, and flexibility. For example, my determination to stay fit comes from a mental image of myself as an old lady who can still climb a mountain, play tennis with my grandchildren, and say yes when invited on an all-day bike ride. Today's children can learn to cultivate their own visions of opportunities unfettered by lack of fitness.

3. The meaning of a physically active lifestyle is misunderstood.

Many people have faulty ideas about exercise that come from the media, especially the fitness market. Following are some important facts:

Movement of any kind makes a difference.

When it comes to exercise, an all-or-nothing mentality is self-defeating. No pain, no gain is a myth, and the notion that only intense aerobic workouts are worth anything leads many people to give up the idea that they could be more fit. An overall reduction in sedentary activities and the addition of even minimal, but routine physical activity (such as twenty minutes of energetic walking per day) can have more significant health benefits than occasional bursts of aerobic exercise. If it works for your child to be actively engaged in sports, dance, or other activities that include a high level of aerobic fitness, that's great. But if none of these are your child's thing, there is still a lot he or she can do to maintain strength, health, and fitness.

Intense competition is not for everyone.

Many adolescents drop out of sports, gymnastics, or dance that they once enjoyed in grade school because pressures to compete take the fun out of it. Kids who just want to have fun with these pastimes too often feel coerced by coaches, parents, or even teammates to try out for higher levels, making recreation stressful for them. You can help your child tune in to the type of participation that fits best for her, rather than resorting to dropping out.

Kids and adults who are not athletically inclined, especially if they are large bodied, need encouragement to be active in ways that leave them feeling successful and that can be an on-going, enjoyable part of their lives. This means success cannot be measured by the same standards of performance used for more physically talented kids. Less-athletic kids are turned off by physical-education classes that grade them on skill level rather than involvement, effort, and personal improvement. Talk to the director of the department if your child feels she cannot be successful in physical education.

Physical activity should be enjoyable.
There are virtually unlimited ways for kids and adults to be active while having fun. As most adults will attest, exercise programs undertaken only to work out, but that are boring and tedious, take too much travel time, or require complicated scheduling are doomed from the start. As role models, the best way to help our kids to value lifelong fitness is to be physically active, doing things we like to do that easily fit into the day. This may require some creative thinking, but the effort is worth it.

If you hate to go to the gym, which I can relate to, then don't go to the gym. On pages 192–94 is a list of ideas to get you up and moving. You and your child can make physical activity an enjoyable part of your routine with the right intention. When your child sees that you make fitness a priority, right along with other self-care, this will send a powerful message that it is an important part of life. The pleasure of active recreation naturally balances the satisfaction of healthy hunger and enjoyment of good food for a high quality life.

Physical activity should balance the other events in our day.
Like everything else in this book, the key is balance. Physical activity should be one part of a well-rounded life, not something that is done excessively or compulsively. For most busy people, it takes a bit of discipline to fit it in, but for a few people, exercise can take on too much of a life of its own. If your child appears to be driven to exercise too much of the time, this may be a symptom of an underlying problem. If talking to her does not seem to help her regain her perspective, you will want to discuss this behavior with a professional.

HELPING KIDS WITH PREJUDICE ABOUT SIZE

Children are sometimes harassed or put down based on size, especially when they join in vigorous activities. Prejudice about weight is wrong. It is usually based on ignorance, but regardless of the reason, weightist attitudes can have long-term damaging effects. Whether your child is fat or thin, help him or her to understand these facts:

• It shows intelligence for everyone to be physically active.

• Weightism is a form of prejudice. It is usually based on ignorance (versus merely meanness), but it is wrong nonetheless.

• Anyone who is the target of prejudice will feel hurt, sad, and probably angry. In any case, they will want it stopped, which is completely justified.

• If a child is the target of prejudice based on size, give this advice:

Don't let it stop you from being physically active.

Look for kids who will support you in feeling good
about being active.

Tell a grown-up who understands that negative teasing
or put-downs of any kind are wrong and who will
do something to prevent it.

FACT: Active teenagers of every size and shape say they feel
better about themselves and their bodies than teenagers who
are not physically active do.

TALKING WITH KIDS

Use the following questions and information as fuel for conversations with your child. Then suggest the Activity Diary on page 195. Your child will probably get more out of this activity if you and others in the family join in it too.

Is it important to be physically active?

Physical activity is very important for health. Whether we are fatter or thinner, if we eat well and are physically active we can be confident our weight is right for us. Physical fitness helps bodies run their best to burn the food we eat and to stay fit.

What is physical activity?

Physical activity means we are awake and moving. This can range from very little movement to a lot. Very little movement is called sedentary and means mostly we are sitting in one place. A lot of movement is called aerobic and means we are moving so much that our body is racing inside and out.

The list below describes the full range of movement that is possible. Ask your child if she can think of activities from her own life that fit each category.

1. Passive sitting—awake but sitting very still. You may be watching something, reading, thinking, talking quietly, or playing a handheld game.
2. Active sitting—sitting, but busy. You may be writing, doing artwork, playing cards, eating, enjoying lively conversation, or playing a more active sitting game in which your upper body is moving.
3. Normal movement—moving about with normal exertion, such as in normal walking, with no rise in heart rate or increase in breathing. You are on your feet, playing, shopping, picking up your room, giving a speech, or attending a class that requires you to move around.
4. Vigorous movement—on the go at a fast pace. You may be walking fast, playing a running game, climbing trees, or riding your bike. This kind of movement includes a significant rise in heart rate and breathing, but these either come in short bursts of time or are a moderate rise sustained for a longer time.
5. Aerobic movement—moving so that your heart is beating very rapidly for an extended time (thirty minutes or more). This might include playing soccer, basketball, or some other sport; dancing hard; distance running; swimming or aerobic walking; skiing; in-line skating; or biking at a fast pace.

Doesn't physical activity just happen as part of life?

The way people live has changed a great deal in the past sixty years. People have always had parts of their day when they were active, such as when they were running and playing with friends, and times when they were sedentary, such as when they were reading or sitting at a desk in school. But until recently, people had to be much more physically active just to stay alive. People had to work with their bodies every day to earn money, get food, have a nice home or quality of life, or move from one part of town to another. Sixty years ago, exercise for the sake of exercise was not something most people had to think about, because they got quite a workout without even knowing it. Now, we have a lot of machines that help us do our work and vehicles to carry us around. Ask your child to think of things that used to be a workout that are no longer necessary for most people. (Examples include chopping wood to burn for heat; shoveling coal; washing laundry by hand and hanging it to dry; routinely walking to find, hunt, or buy food, visit friends or relatives, make a pilgrimage, or go to school; digging a garden; sweeping floors; beating rugs; sewing clothes; carrying water.)

As a rule, today's lifestyles do not require significant physical activity. If choices aren't made to limit sedentary entertainment or free-time options and to look for daily opportunities that include movement, a serious deficit in physical activity is very likely to occur by default.

In addition to machines that do much of our work, many new forms of entertainment that involve sitting have come about in the past sixty years. Today, people are more sedentary than ever before. Take turns with your child naming sedentary activities that you enjoy or participate in. See how many you can think of.

What happens when bodies are sedentary?

Our bodies have changed a lot since humans lived in caves. For example, we have a lot less hair than we used to, and we are much taller, bigger, and smarter. In some ways, however, we haven't changed. Our muscles still require physical use to keep them healthy and strong. Since machines and vehicles have eliminated a lot of the activity that used to take care of this, muscles that are not well used, including the heart muscle, become weak. When this happens, our heart must work much harder to circulate the blood that keeps the rest of our body working properly, and our risk for many diseases increases.

Another way that humans have not changed is that we get just as hungry now as when we were more active. Food provides energy to keep our bodies going, and the more active we are, the more energy we need. If we are less active but have the same amount of hunger to satisfy, our bodies naturally have to store the unused energy as fat. This is particularly true for people who are born with a slow metabolism to begin with. (These are the people who were most likely to survive a long winter when food was scarce.) While some people will always be fatter and others are born to be slim, this drop in our physical activity has resulted in many people gaining more weight than is healthy for them.

To solve this problem, experts have agreed there are two things people should do to know for sure that they are healthy and to feel confident that their weight is right for them:

- Satisfy hunger completely with enough good, wholesome food at regular meals.
- Limit sedentary entertainment, and be sure to include time for plenty of physical activity every day.

If you make these two choices a priority in your life, you can trust that you are achieving two important goals: (1) you are doing your part to keep your body healthy and fit, and (2) you are discovering the weight that is right for you.

What do you have to do to be physically active?

Playing or working hard in ways that get your heart pumping every single day is the best for great health. But this is not the only way to be physically active. You might play in a sport, jog, or work out in a gym, but you could also stand on your head, have a pillow fight, run around with the dog, in-line skate, cook dinner and do the dishes, swing, ride a bike, dance in your room, play drums, or walk instead of riding in a car—just about anything that gets you on your feet and moving.

Here are a few common myths about physical activity:

No pain, no gain.
Some people think the only way to develop physical fitness is to work out to the point of muscle pain and burning lungs.
Fact: Getting your heart pumping for at least thirty minutes most days is something your body will thank you for. But *any* vigorous movement that lasts for ten minutes or longer will improve your health. Too much sitting is the *biggest* problem. How much time do you currently spend on sedentary entertainment options? Think about how many hours of free time you have per day. Could you limit how much of this time is spent sitting? The Activity Diary on page 195 will help you analyze this more carefully.

Physical activity is for people who are athletic or in sports.
Fact: Physical activity is for everyone. You can support your

health and feel confident in your weight if you are on the move, doing active things you like to do throughout the day, every day. Many kids who are not in sports sit for hours at school followed by homework and then television or computer or electronic games in the evening. Such sedentary entertainment should be limited to allow time for physical activity.

Fatter people can't be physically active.

Fact: What if we said, "People who aren't good at math can't learn to add and subtract?" "People who are short can't play basketball." "People who are tall can't ride in sports cars." This is the kind of thing we are saying if we say, "Fatter people cannot be physically active." The truth is, everyone should be physically active. This myth assumes fatter people are not or cannot be in shape. Some people who are very thin are not fit at all, and some people who are fat are extremely fit. You cannot tell how a person eats by how they look, and you cannot tell how active they are either. Everyone should get plenty of activity every day.

STAYING ACTIVE

Adults who have an active lifestyle have found the following tips helpful. Many of the tips apply to kids too, but never expect kids to stay active in ways that are not also fun for them. If your kids have been inactive, it may take some time to discover vigorous play activities they enjoy.

• It is the automatic nature of behaviors that make them a routine part of our lifestyle. In the same way that you brush your teeth daily whether you feel like it or not, plan to be active every day without asking, "Do I feel like it today?" Let it become part of how you live.

• To include physical activity in your routine, you have to allot time for it. Just as you set aside time for meals, hygiene, work, friends, and quiet time, you may need to have a protected time slot for physical activity. Formally schedule this into your day. Combining fitness activities with other enjoyable events can be time efficient.

• Pair an activity with another natural break in the day, such as first thing in the morning, during lunch, or before or after dinner.

• Things that are part of our lifestyle become part of our identity. Decide to make "I'm an active, fit person" part of your identity—among the top ten things you would say to describe yourself.

• If you have been sedentary, start at your current level of fitness (which may mean a slow walk around the block) and work up to thirty minutes (or more) of movement (such as fast walking) that gets your heart pumping.

• For out-of-shape kids, an increase in activity might be as simple as walking or biking somewhere instead of getting a ride (with or without you, depending on age). Kids will only continue an activity if they enjoy it, get into the competitiveness of a game, see it as a means to connect socially, or as a means to more freedom/independence.

• If you live in a climate with cold winters, plan to buy long underwear and be active outdoors year-round once you have strengthened your heart and lungs to an aerobic level. An aerobic walk will keep you warm even at below-zero temperatures if you are dressed in layers and have your head covered. Get shoes with good traction for icy ground and some of the new high-tech underwear for warmth. Take pride in not letting the weather stop you! ⟶

• Put on the music and dance in your living room (alone or with a partner). Do it for ten minutes, if that's all you have time or endurance for, or until you are bored.

• Bike, in-line skate, cross-country ski, or swim in a nearby lake or neighborhood pool.

• Play tennis, dribble a soccer ball, shoot baskets in the park, play catch, or join a recreational sports team.

• Garden or do other yard work, clean the house at a vigorous pace, sweep the driveway, wash the car.

• Play active games (inside or out).

• Offer to walk your neighbor's dog.

• "No fuss" is a requirement for most things that become part of our lifestyle. What if every time you showered, you had to hunt for the soap? Keep appropriate shoes, clothes, and equipment handy.

THE ACTIVITY PYRAMID

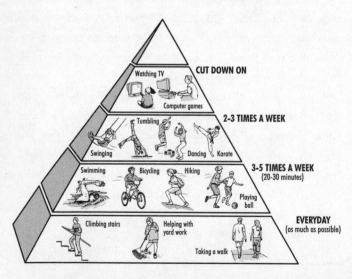

BODY LIFT

ACTIVITY DIARY

Does your child balance the amount of time spent sitting with enough movement? Does she get her heart pumping? Help your child find out by keeping an Activity Diary. Take a look at the sample diary on page 196 to see how it's done. Then photocopy the Activity Diary on page 197 to keep track of activity habits for several days. Each participant will need one of the Activity Diary sheets for each day, or seven sheets. You can guesstimate the time you spent on different types of activities to the nearest fifteen minutes. Use your estimates to fill in the chart. For non–school days, have your child combine the divided blocks of time into simply morning and afternoon.

After completing the Activity Diary sheets for several days, compare your results to the recommendations in the Activity Pyramid. Ask your child the following questions:

- Did you get plenty of movement (walking, taking the stairs, playing outside, or active indoor play) every day?
- Did you do an aerobic activity for thirty minutes at least three times a week?
- Did you move vigorously for thirty minutes or more on many days?
- Do you think you're getting enough physical activity?
- If not, how can you fit more activity into your life?

SAMPLE ACTIVITY DIARY

Passive sitting: Sitting still, absorbed and focused; TV, computer games, reading

Active sitting: Sitting, but busy; writing, artwork, playing cards, eating

Normal movement: Up and moving; normal walking, building an indoor fort, doing dishes, shopping

Vigorous movement: On the go; swinging, climbing, hide and seek, playing catch, heavy chores

Aerobic movement: Any activity that makes your heart race for several minutes or more

	PASSIVE SITTING	ACTIVE SITTING	NORMAL MOVEMENT	VIGOROUS MOVEMENT	AEROBIC MOVEMENT
BEFORE SCHOOL		petted cat—15 min. ate—15 min. rode bus—15 min.	shower—15 min. got dressed—15 min.	did cartwheels at bus stop—15 min.	
SCHOOLDAY MORNING	read and listened—30 min.	work at desk—1 hour	library—30 min.	Phys-ed—15 min.	Phys-ed—15 min.
LUNCH PERIOD		lunch—30 min	walked and talked—15 min.	played 4-square—15 min.	
SCHOOLDAY AFTERNOON	read and listened; saw video—1¼ hour	writing a test—30 min. worked in small group—30 min.	choir practice—30 min. walking—15 min.	spelling bee (very nervous!)—15 min.	
AFTER SCHOOL UNTIL DINNER	TV—1 hour	rode bus—15 min. homework—30 min.	walked dog—15 min.	soccer warm-up—30 min.	played soccer—45 min.
AFTER DINNER UNTIL BED	computer game—30 min. read—15 min.	dinner—30 min. artwork—15 min. talked on phone—15 min. piano—30 min.	walked dog—15 min. did dishes—15 min. played with sister—30 min.		
TOTALS	3½ hours	5½ hours	3¾ hours	1½ hour	60 min.

ACTIVITY DIARY

Passive sitting: Sitting still, absorbed and focused; TV, computer games, reading
Active sitting: Sitting, but busy; writing, artwork, playing cards, eating
Normal movement: Up and moving; normal walking, building an indoor fort, doing dishes, shopping
Vigorous movement: On the go; swinging, climbing, hide and seek, playing catch, heavy chores
Aerobic movement: Any activity that makes your heart race for several minutes or more

	PASSIVE SITTING	ACTIVE SITTING	NORMAL MOVEMENT	VIGOROUS MOVEMENT	AEROBIC MOVEMENT
BEFORE SCHOOL					
SCHOOLDAY MORNING					
LUNCH PERIOD					
SCHOOLDAY AFTERNOON					
AFTER SCHOOL UNTIL DINNER					
AFTER DINNER UNTIL BED					
TOTAL					

Also available at www.bodyimagehealth.org

BODY-ESTEEM AFFIRMATIONS

When your child understands this essential lesson, she will embrace statements like these:

- To be strong and healthy, it's important to get some exercise every day.
- My body can do a lot of things.
- I am physically active most days.
- There are lots of ways to be active besides sports or working out in a gym.
- Even if TV and electronic games are fun, I will make sure I also spend my time in activities that keep me strong and fit.
- I am physically active and eat well, so I am confident of my weight.

Lesson 9:
Sold on Looks:
The Influence of Mass Media

By carefully and purposefully manipulating our view of reality, mass media plays a significant role in defining what is normal and desirable today. As such, it is a mighty force in our lives and the lives of our children. Unfortunately, normal and desirable have come to mean purchasing the "right" stuff, in order to have the "right" image, which in turn should make us happy. As many young teens will tell you, the value of inner beauty seems to pale when compared to this promise— which can supposedly be purchased at "stores everywhere!"

When we try to teach our children that they are more than how they look, we have to understand that our message is going to meet with very stiff competition. Chances are good that every day our kids will hear a conflicting set of seductive, powerful claims telling them that it's not who they are, but how they are packaged that really counts. Making matters worse, this message hits our kids hardest precisely when they begin to separate from us and turn to the wider culture for guidance.

Many of us would like to see a change in media messages that make it so hard to raise our kids with healthy perspectives. For readers who want to take action, I've listed groups that work on behalf of this goal in appendix D on page 241. But change takes time, and our kids are being affected now. It is therefore vital that we help children learn how to interpret and resist the virtual reality of advertising by teaching them how marketing

→ strategically creates *images* (that may not be what they seem)

➜ in order to provoke *feelings*
    ➜ that result in a perceived *need*
       ➜ which can best be met by a *product.*

You'll also teach your child to translate the most common photo advertisement "language." A typical translation would be:

➜ Look at this happy, successful, popular, and appealing model. Clearly she's got what it takes.
    ➜ Compared to this model, you are deficient or missing something.
       ➜ In order to have what it takes, you need improvement.
         ➜ You need [our product]!

THE MARKETING OF NEW STANDARDS FOR GOOD LOOKS

State-of-the-art mass-marketing campaigns have made it relatively easy to persuade large numbers of people that they

---

THE PERFECT WOMAN

Most female models in ads are extraordinarily beautiful, sophisticated, sleek, and very, very slim. They have only smooth lines and no fat. Their clothes hang perfectly, without a lump or bulge. Skin is completely clear, without a bump, wrinkle, or blemish. Mouths are perfectly drawn and colored, eyes are bright and even, with long, silky lashes. Every hair shines. Only 3 women in 100 naturally have the body type and look of the models used in most advertising. By comparison, this has made a lot of women worry that they are too fat and that their natural size and shape are not acceptable.

should discard former standards of appearance and embrace new ones, even when the new standards are not realistic or good for most of us. Standards that define who and what is good-looking have changed dramatically in a very short time.

It is one thing when mass media defines what's in and out when it comes to fashion, makeup, and hair care. But the use of prototype fashion models to sell any and all products, ranging from cars and toothpaste to alcohol and plumbing supplies, has completely redefined what is considered to be an acceptable body size and shape for ordinary people. The message is, "If you don't look like this model, you must not be trying hard enough (but our product will help!)." The average American woman, who is five foot four inches and weighs 144 pounds, now compares her body to that of the average American model, who is five foot eleven and weighs

---

THE PERFECT MAN

Male models in ads are strikingly handsome. Often they have intense eyes that look cool, detached, and faraway, or they seem to look right through you. The take-charge eyes above strong chins and straight noses let you know these men are tough, in control of what's happening, and clearly have it all. Their bodies are chiseled into broad shoulders supported by slim hips. If they are bare-chested, we see lots of developed muscles, including a "six-pack" over their abdomen. Advertisers are learning that men can also feel insecure about their looks when enough advertisements present unusually well-developed male bodies. It can take hours per day of working out for men to develop their muscles in this way. While they are overall more muscular than females, males also are naturally predisposed to vary in fatness and thinness.

117 pounds. In 1954 the percentage of weight difference between the average American woman and the average American model was just 4 percent; today it is 25 percent. Symbolizing beauty for all, today's models represent a body type that is natural for fewer than 3 percent of the female population. The Barbie doll, who would be grotesque if she came to life, is still idolized by young girls who are not clear she is a fantasy. Teenagers describe the ideal girl as five foot seven inches tall, weighing 110 pounds, with blue eyes and long blonde hair. No wonder women feel fat and insecure!

The male wish to be seen as attractive has been exploited less, but surveys suggest this is changing. Studies show that, surrounded by a growing number of images of ideally handsome men with the chiseled-body look, men are feeling increasingly deficient in comparison.

THE MARKETING OF NEW IDEAS FOR SHAPING THE BODY

Many people do not recognize that today's standard for size and shape would never have gained so much ground without the companion belief that anyone can have the requisite lean body through diet and exercise. Advertisements promoting the latest weight-loss diet or quick-fix to "Lose weight while you sleep," "Burn ugly fat and flatten your tummy," or "Double your metabolism with no extra effort!" are everyday fare. Book racks are bulging with titles promising any buyer she can be *Thin for Life*. It is actually this combination package (the idolization of thinness plus the belief that through the right effort anyone can achieve it) that directly or indirectly causes most of the body-image, eating, and weight problems seen today. Many countries throughout the world produce media images of high-fashion models, but do not have significant body dissatisfaction and eating problems in their population. The difference appears to be the absence of the diet mentality in these cultures. As a result, people view models chosen for their slender appearances without feeling they should try to imitate them. Surely this reflects a more gracious acceptance of our biological limitations and an appreciation of real people in real bodies demonstrating healthy body esteem.

Even a brief (twenty-minute) intensive exposure to images of typical fashion models provokes an immediate drop in self-esteem.

The American economy may have benefited from the manufactured belief that it is necessary to worry and work endlessly to reshape body size, but much has been lost. We are richer, but do not look any better, and clearly we feel worse. Many adults try to laugh off their appearance insecurities in order to cope. But when it comes to our children, it doesn't seem funny. Deep down, we know how much time and energy our self-consciousness has cost us. Kids can develop more realistic body images and maintain healthier expectations about looks if we prepare them to understand destructive media messages.

THE MARKETING OF NEW WAYS TO THINK OF FOOD

Thanks to mass marketing, food has a new purpose: entertainment. By presenting supersized portions of delicious-tasting, high-calorie but low-nutrient food as normal eating and by making it widely available at cheap prices everywhere, marketers have created a generation of children and adults who don't seem to know that a primary purpose of eating is to provide our bodies with nutrients. I know a lot of people who won't eat food that does not have high entertainment value.

Many kids think potato chips count as vegetables. Toys, such as the McDonald's Barbie, or action figures that are actually containers for candy, advertise food. Most children under the age of eight are not able to understand that ads for these products are not created with their interest at heart, but rather to make money.

THE MARKETING OF NEW VALUES FOR LIFE: HAPPINESS CAN BE PURCHASED

It is hard to fathom the hidden purposes of marketing, particularly when it comes to the campaigns that are aimed directly at children. At the annual Golden Marbles Awards (the equivalent of the Academy Awards for advertising) held on Wall Street, ad agencies celebrate the cleverest and most effective ways to "capture children's minds" and to "own kids" (quotes from guest speakers). At conventions for marketers, presenters openly state their intent to play on kids' vulnerabilities in declarations such as, "Remember, all kids want to do is fit in. Brand them when they're babies!" The two primary products sold to children are food and toys, but marketing of clothing and makeup aimed at teaching preschoolers to be consumers of the right look is on the rise.

Such marketers seem to be willing to discount children's well-being and physical health for commercial gain. Not only are children directly affected, but ads teach kids how to nag parents into purchasing "got to have it" commodities and treats as well. Marketing makes a parent's job tougher every day. Other countries have laws to protect children from this kind of manipulation. In Scandinavia it is assumed that advertising to kids should be restricted. Sweden and Norway specifically prohibit television ads directed at children below twelve years of age. TV commercials for toys are banned in Greece until 10 P.M. and it is forbidden to broadcast commercials during children's programs in Belgium, as well as during the five minutes before and after them. In contrast, in the United States, parents have the added burden of teaching children to resist the continual barrage of messages that conflict with more substantial values.

VIEWER BEWARE

A new media trick is to take the best parts of two or more models and put them together in one picture to make one ideal model. Legs may belong to one model, the face to another. Might this be true for some of the ads you have looked at? Movies sometimes do this as well, showing one actress's body and another's face. Models and movie stars even feel bad about themselves when they compare how they look in real life to their enhanced photos. Remember, media pictures are created to get you to buy the product. Do not compare yourself to these unrealistic photos.

TALKING WITH KIDS

Your child's readiness for media literacy will depend in part on her age and will progress as she grows. Use this section as a guide for conversation with your child.

Media literacy

With preschool children, you can begin to help them to distinguish between the purpose of an ad (to sell something) and the entertainment value of a program. Explain that the people who made the commercials want us to see the ad and buy the product so they can make money. Even three- to five-year-old children can understand that advertisers want to make the product look more appealing than it is in real life. This introduces your child to the concept of manufactured images, in contrast to photos of real people and things.

For kids in early elementary school you can adapt the "How Stories Are Told by Pictures in Advertising" activity on pages 211–14 to raise awareness about what marketers want to make children believe about the product. You can say something like, "It seems like the people who made that cereal want you to believe you will win at soccer every time if you eat their cereal. And then everyone on the team will want to be your friend, and you will be happy forever! Do you think that would happen in real life?"

When your child is in the upper elementary grades, teach her that understanding sales tactics (and the entertainment that is sponsored by advertising) is an important life skill, similar to money management. If your child has already studied media literacy in school or elsewhere, you can build on or reinforce this. Share the following child-friendly information with your child.

Why do looks matter more to some people than others?

Humans have always been interested in looks. Throughout history people have taken pleasure in decorating their bodies, dressing up, and looking nice. Still, most people have understood that happiness does not come from superficial appearances and that how we look is not the most important part of a person. That is why sayings like these are well known: "You can't judge a book by its cover." "Beauty is only skin deep."

In spite of this wisdom, looks somehow seem to matter a lot to some people today. Americans spend many billions of dollars each year on how they look. With your child, brainstorm a list of things that are purchased only for the sake of our appearance: trendy clothing, stylish shoes, makeup, skin-care products, hair-care products, jewelry, diet products, diet/weight-loss books, fashion magazines, cosmetic surgery, and so on.

Most of us enjoy looking nice. But if looks are not all that important, why do we spend so much time and effort attempting to improve our appearance? Surveys of Americans tell us that people worry about looks a lot more now than they did forty years ago—much more than any culture ever has before. Why is this? Another saying offers us a clue: "One picture is worth a thousand words."

Changes in people's feelings and opinions about looks have occurred in the past forty years because of pictures.

Pictures, pictures, everywhere!

Until the 1950s, people mostly had other ordinary people to look at in their everyday life. At that time, there were very few fashion magazines, no TV, and just a few movies. It was fairly rare to see many pictures of extraordinarily "good-looking" people. While people were interested in glamorous or handsome movie stars, entertainers, famous athletes, or fashion models, most people did not compare their own looks to them.

In the 1950s, televisions became affordable, and the average person was able to buy one for home use. With this new technology, suddenly there was a huge increase in how many glamorous people ordinary people saw every day. This grew and grew. By the 1960s, TV, movies, magazines, newspapers, billboards, and, in particular, the advertising that paid for all of these were presenting pictures of carefully chosen, unusually good-looking models and entertainment stars everywhere. People saw more pictures in a few months than most people had previously seen in a whole lifetime. If "one picture is worth a thousand words," can you imagine all the stories these hundreds and thousands of pictures told?

How are looks defined as "good"?

The standard for "good-looking" has changed many times throughout history. Prior to mass media (TV, movies, magazines), fads and fashions changed very slowly. It could take a hundred years or more for a style of clothing or hairstyle to come and go. What was considered good looking often depended on what people needed to survive. For example, fatter bodies were desired when food was in short supply, which was true throughout much of history.

With mass-media advertising, new ideas about looks can be shown to the whole population in just a few weeks. What is in today may be out in a year, rather than a century or two. With your child, try to think of some fads that have come and gone in your lifetime.

We now know that when we see many pictures of people, all with one way of looking, it can have a big effect on how we define good looks. When such pictures surround us all the time—in magazines, on billboards, in the movies, on TV, in store windows—it is natural to decide that the model's look is what is normal. After a while, it seems that anyone who doesn't look that way is not good-looking.

Advertisers know that if you want to look like their models, this increases the chance that you will want to buy the product that is shown with the models. While it is not realistic, we can be tricked into feeling we have to have what the models have in order to be attractive or liked. We compare ourselves and get worried that we do not look as good. This is a formula for feeling bad. All of a sudden, we feel we have to put a lot of time and money into improving our looks.

Understanding advertising

Businesses spend millions of dollars creating clever ways to attract us to their advertisements. The cost is worth it to them if they can succeed in making millions of us buy their product.

Advertisers could use words to tell us about their products, but most ads include a picture. Pictures tell stories that leave a big impression on us. Advertisers work very hard to make sure we feel we *have to have* the product they are selling.

Advertisers hope to awaken our natural wish to be special when we look at images of beautiful people. Think twice. Do you believe that the way to be special is through trying to have a certain look? Too often people can be tricked into worrying too much about looks. As your child gets older, it's natural for her to become more and more interested in looking nice. She may want to feel attractive and enjoy fun clothes and hairstyles. When this happens, you can remind her to be smart and take care not to let the stories told in advertising trick her into a formula for feeling bad.

BODY LIFT

READING ADVERTISEMENT STORIES

You can do this activity with your child alone or with a group of her or his friends. (Be sure to get other parents' permission.) First collect several photo advertisements from magazines, newspapers, or flyers. The ads you choose should represent the following four categories:

1. A few ads that include typical slim and beautiful or buff and handsome models selling products designed to produce a look (clothing fashions, makeup, skin-care and hair-care products)

2. Ads that have little to do with appearance and are being presented by these same typically ideal models (cars, lawn mowers, orange juice, cigarettes)

3. Two or more ads selling diet products or plans. These should also include photos of men or women. Be sure at least one of the ads you use has outrageously unrealistic claims.

4. Finally, a few typical ads that present high-sugar, low-nutrient treats as if they were nutritious meal or snack options.

Begin by simply looking at all the photos you have selected, reading the words, and describing the photo: "Here's a lady with a big smile and shiny red hair selling toothpaste." "Here's a happy-looking teen and her friends modeling jeans." Then use the following guide to determine the stories being told in the ads.

HOW STORIES ARE TOLD BY PICTURES
IN ADVERTISING

The story line . . .	answers the question . . .
Our product is for you!	Whose attention does this ad hope to attract? **Examples:** You are a mom, teen, pet lover, girl, boy, dancer, athlete, gardener, romantic, cook, etc.
See the model . . .	How does the model look? What is she doing, and how does she appear to be feeling? **Examples:** She or he is beautiful or handsome, and very slim or muscular. Also happy, popular, secure, healthy, successful, fun-loving, in charge, etc.
The model's appearance reminds you of something you want.	The photo wakes your desire for something. **Examples:** You want joy, money, health, adventure, friends and love, etc
You wonder: How does your life compare with the model's?	Do you have what the model appears to have? **Examples:** She or he appears to have everything it takes to be happy. You could be or are missing something. You are or could be deficient or inadequate in some way.
You want what it appears the model has.	What do you want? **Examples:** **Beauty:** great hair, teeth, eyes, skin, less fat, great legs, big muscles, smooth hands, long fingernails, sexy feet, young skin, the right look **Popularity:** attractiveness, sparkle, pizzazz, "what it takes" **Power:** control, money, wisdom, fame, prestige, the right image **Purpose:** a cause, an identity, romance, the meaning of life, escape from it all **Balance:** time, health, comfort, peace of mind, safety
You need	What will fulfill your needs? **Our product!**

Interpret the story line for several different products. Be sure to look for small details that the advertiser included to make the story more convincing (for example, facial expressions, postures, props). You can have fun with this. The more out-

rageous the ad, the better. Point out that many ads selling different products have a common story line:

> *You need something. In fact, if you compare what you know*
> *about your life to what you see in these models, you know*
> *there is a lot you could improve on. See how this model is*
> *completely happy, healthy, and in control? Without a doubt,*
> *she is having a better life than you are. You can see this from*
> *how amazingly good she looks. If you buy her product,*
> *maybe you and your life will be more like hers.*

FOLLOW-UP QUESTIONS

After you translate the story lines in your ads, discuss these
questions:

- How do you feel when you look at the models in the ads?
  Are the ads appealing?
- Would you be tempted to buy the product? Why or why not?
- Do the pictures give you any ideas about how people should
  look?
- Will the products make you look like the models?
- Will the products make you happy?
- How do you feel if you compare yourself to the models in
  the pictures?
- Do you think you could look like the models in the pictures?
  Why or why not?
- How much would it cost to try? If you spent the money,
  how would you feel if you still didn't look like the model?

You and your child can make a game of translating the hidden
messages on covers of magazines in stores, commenting on
the images of bigger-than-life models in store windows at the
mall, or discussing television advertisements that portray
"ideal" looks as part of the sales tactic. Take care not to choose

ads selling or portraying sexually suggestive themes that might embarrass your child—although for older teens it is effective to study this advertising agenda.

BODY-ESTEEM AFFIRMATIONS

When your child understands this essential lesson, she will embrace statements like these:

- I am wise to the fact that advertisers want to persuade us that we have to have something to be happy—and then offer their product as the best way to fill that need.
- If an advertisement makes me feel I'm not quite good enough, I'll remember this is part of the sales tactic.
- Hardly anyone looks as perfect as the models in advertisements. I will be careful not to compare myself to them.
- Looks are nice, but deeper qualities are more valuable when it comes to real happiness.
- I can enjoy pictures of beautiful people and still feel confident about myself.

Lesson 10:
Choosing Healthy Role Models

"Everyone wants to be my friend because I have the coolest clothes." —six-year-old girl

Adolescents face big challenges as they begin to define themselves as young men and women. Taking the first steps toward independence from parents generates tremendous excitement, but at the same time, a sense of insecurity that is natural, given their inexperience. There are so many firsts at this age! Eager to try their wings, but still needing a lot of reassurance, preteens and adolescents transfer their huge dependency needs onto their peers. The only solace for anxiety seems to come from being included, which makes fitting in feel absolutely essential at this time. To avoid all risk of being left out, most kids become enormously invested in not appearing different. It is at this precarious time that many adolescents feel forced to choose between who they really are and trying to be like everyone else. Unfortunately, it is less often who they are than who they can appear to be that seems to matter.

At this stage, a child's choice of role models can be critical. Exploiting this vulnerability, the strategic use of crafted role models has become a common marketing strategy, especially to target girls. For example, when it comes to ads portraying men, Guess's executive for advertising, Paul Marciano, said he is proud that his ads "use real men—real cowboys, ranchers, truck drivers, and an actual matador. My field is day-to-day street life. I don't want to create fake pictures." In contrast, his ads portraying women are another matter. In that regard, Marciano said, "We always use models. It's difficult to find real women who fit what we're trying to say. Real women, they aren't as cooperative as real men." With over $12 billion spent on advertising to children per year, our daughters thus learn to strive for the "right" way to look and feel—rather than to look for role models who personify who they really are.

Boys also struggle in adolescence to learn what it takes to fit in. The standards and options, however, appear to be more flexible for boys, and the risks less extreme. Boys may be just as unhappy if they perceive they don't have the right look or personality, but it appears they are more likely to maintain perspective and understand appearance is only one aspect of who they are, not the sum total. What males *do*, versus how they look, takes precedence. When boys' efforts don't produce the desired results, they are more likely to focus their energy on another area in which they can succeed, rather than trying to make themselves over at any cost.

THE NEED FOR POSITIVE ROLE MODELS

We understand it is developmentally normal for kids to choose role models, clothing, and fads that separate them and their peers from their parents. But it can be hard for adults to understand the cruel and self-destructive extremes that adolescents may resort to today. How can parents intervene to encourage the choice of role models that will enhance rather than detract from our children's body esteem?

CONSIDER THE UGLY DUCKLING

Sometimes a question from a simple children's story can help. In this old, familiar story, a stray egg somehow ends up in the nest of a mother duck. It hatches and is judged to be an ugly duckling, which is then ostracized by the other ducks. She finally runs away and grows into a beautiful swan. What if the ugly duckling had stayed with the ducks, accepting a standard that heaped scorn on her own appearance? This, of course, is what many children learn to do: to go along year after year, embracing a standard that can only result in feeling bad. If our child was the swan in *The Ugly Duckling*, we would want to teach those ducks a thing or two about their ignorant, unfair, and cruel judgments. But our first job as parents is to lead our swans with this guiding lesson: Find those with whom you can feel good about who you are. This message is the heart of this lesson and this book.

TALKING WITH KIDS

Reminisce with your child about *The Ugly Duckling*, or read it together if you haven't already. It is a wonderful story, with an important message. As you read or remember this story, consider these questions together with your child:

- What if the swan had stayed with the ducks?
- How did you feel when the swan left the ducks and went off alone? Who decides what is the right way to look or the wrong way?
- Does it matter to what or to whom we compare ourselves? If apples compared themselves to oranges, how would they feel about being apples?
- Have you ever felt like the ugly duckling? What did you do when you felt this way?

Preferences versus judgments

Ask your child: How would you feel if someone said to you in a nasty voice,

- That shirt is ugly.
- I can't believe you'd wear your hair like that.
- That radio station plays stupid music.
- You're too short to play basketball. Fat people like you can't do ballet. Skinny kids like you can't play football.
- Your friend is a nerdy dork.

Point out that these statements are judgments. Judgments determine something is good or bad, or that this way is right and that is wrong. Judgments say this is cool and that is not cool. Share with your child a time when someone made a negative judgment about you or about something you owned. Ask if that's ever happened to him or her.

Now explain that these statements express preferences:

- I like this shirt better than that one.
- I prefer boys with short hair, but that's just me.
- I like pop music more than country-western.
- I like having tall people on my basketball team.
- I don't really understand people who like computers.

Preferences are different from one person to another because everybody's different. For example, some people prefer blue, and some red, while others prefer green or yellow or turquoise. This keeps the world interesting. Preferences do not determine that one thing is good or right while anything else is bad or wrong. There is room for people to have different preferences without anyone feeling bad.

Sometimes things that start out as preferences can turn into judgments. Fads and fashions are this way. Fads can start out as fun—something to do or wear that can bring together anyone who likes that fad. For example, if some kids wanted to wear the school colors every Friday, anyone could be part of that fad, if they wanted to. If they didn't, it wouldn't matter. Most fads come and go. They're cool. They don't hurt anyone. They make life interesting.

Problems arise when people who don't go along with a fad are judged as stupid, uncool, dorky, ugly, etc. When fads and fashions become judgments this can hurt.

What if what's cool doesn't work for someone? What if, like the ugly duckling, the cool way to look just isn't how a person looks? What if someone cannot go along with the latest style or fad, or way of doing things, and still be who he is? Maybe he doesn't like the latest fad. Maybe he's not good at it or doesn't believe in it, or maybe it means acting or looking a certain way that just doesn't fit him. This happens to everyone at some time.

Kids have a strong need to belong. If a child is worried that she might be judged if she exposes her true self, she may hide who she is in hopes of being included.

If your child finds herself feeling pressured to be something or do something that isn't right for her, encourage her to look for people with whom she can feel good about herself. It can help to have role models who reflect who we are deep inside. Everyone has role models. You can help your child to think about the qualities she admires most in a person and to choose realistic role models who will support her in becoming the best that she can be.

BODY LIFT
CHOOSING ROLE MODELS

People we admire often become role models for us. Have your child think of two people she admires and might choose as role models. At least one should be someone she knows personally. The other may be someone she has read or heard about. She should know more than one characteristic of her role model. For example, she may admire a famous athlete, but if she only knows she is a great athlete and nothing more, that would not be adequate.

Now ask your child to list on a blank piece of paper at least five things about each of these people that she admires and would like to model. If she cannot think of at least five things, she should choose a different person. Encourage her to consider deeper qualities in a role model, not just what she sees on the surface. What does the person believe in? How does the person act?

Help your child consider if she would feel happy and strong allowing herself to follow in the footsteps of the role models she chose, or if she would feel uncomfortable in any way. This activity offers a rich opportunity for you to share stories with your child about the people in your life, past and present, who have influenced you. Your child may even benefit from hearing about people you once admired who may have lead you to betray your true self. Balance this by mentioning diverse people, including some whom your child knows, who currently inspire you to be the best friend, worker, neighbor, community member, and parent that you can be. Be sure to point out that these real-life role models come in all sizes.

BODY-ESTEEM AFFIRMATIONS

When your child has learned the essential message of this lesson, she will strongly relate to affirmations like the ones below:

- It helps to have role models you admire for things deep inside.
- People are different. That doesn't mean they are better or worse.
- I know what's right and what isn't right for me.
- I can stay true to what I like even if others don't think it's cool.
- Fads and fashions can be fun, but if they are used to judge people, they can be hurtful and harmful.
- You have to be who you are on the inside, even if others don't understand or like it.
- I will look for friends who help me feel good about myself.

AFTERWORD

THE VIEW FROM
YOUR KITCHEN TABLE

I wrote this book to help parents teach their children to resist
the body-image, eating, and weight problems that are so
prevalent in the American culture. I know that many people
feel alone and uncertain about what to do about these concerns. It can help to reduce the sense of isolation when people discover that most Americans today struggle with some
aspect of body image, eating, and weight. But learning that
these problems are rapidly spreading around the world and
have been identified as a serious world health concern makes
it even clearer that they are insidious and should be stopped.
If you are like most people, such information fuels your determination to provide a healthy model for the children clos-
est to you. With this in mind, ending this book with a glance
at the global picture seems the right thing to do.

THE GLOBAL VIEW

In today's morning paper I read this headline: Anorexia Takes Hold in India. Dieting for weight loss is not a behavior one generally associates with countries like India. How could restrictive eating get a foothold in an environment where up to 60 percent of the population still struggles to get enough to eat? Surely any woman who adopted the Western ultrathin ideal would be scorned. Traditional beauty in India, as in most developing countries, is embodied in a healthy woman with a rounded figure—reflecting the value that it is good to be well fed. But according to today's news, "the arrival of cable television, Western fashions and films in India has given financially comfortable teenagers the idea that thin is beautiful." Similarly, unhealthy, unrealistic body image expectations are a growing problem in many developing countries such as Mexico, Argentina, the Philippines, and many Asian countries where Western beauty ideals and the diet mentality have recently been imported.

Along with the thinness schema, Western culture is also exporting the fast-food industry. In India, for example, while half of the population earns less than one dollar per day (and is thereby excluded from indulging), urban middle- and upper-class families have reportedly been seduced by the introduction of this new, tasty, low-nutrient, high-energy fare. The result, as you might guess, is reflected in another recent headline, India Faces a Weight Problem. Apparently Western fast food, increased sedentary entertainment options, and the thin ideal have all very quickly made their mark on the affluent in a big way. The result is what you might expect after reading this book: the self-defeating cycle of restrictive dieting followed by fast food bonanzas then back to dieting again. As this second news report states, "It looks like the Indian weight-loss industry has a healthy future."

Many countries have followed in the footsteps of the United States in the last decade with a rise in negative body image, as well as dieting disorders and overweight. The good news, according to the BBC, is that already "there is growing agreement that something has to change." But in the United States, where this problem developed over forty years ago, most health and governmental leaders still cannot see the big picture when it comes to understanding what change will be effective. The missing perspective?

Excessive weight and obesity, values about eating and physical activity, the pervasive thin ideal, and weightism are not separate concerns but all part of one interrelated problem.

Currently in mainstream health education we have one model to prevent unhealthy fatness, a different model to prevent dieting and eating disorders, a third model to encourage body esteem, and a fourth to eliminate prejudicial weightist attitudes. When these models conflict, which they usually do, or are counterproductive, which they almost always are, chaos prevails. Such is the current state of affairs. The only solution is a single model that addresses all of these concerns simultaneously.

What does this mean for you and your child?

It means that preventing your children or teens from developing a restrictive eating disorder does *not* mean they should follow today's popular style of eating whatever/whenever, and accept unhealthy fatness if that is the end result.

Yet many of today's kids and adults see it in this all-or-nothing way.

It means that preventing compulsive overeating, binge eating, or simply too much carefree consumption does not mean bigger and better diet programs, or urging people to use more willpower to restrict calories. Yet the majority of Americans (even physicians) still believe dieting is the only way out.

It means that the solution for the injustice of weightism is not angry defiance about healthy eating and lifestyle choices. Yet many naturally fatter people don't know how else to fight back.

What those of us in the trenches have learned, and the research now affirms, is that a holistic approach with *health at any size* as the goal is the only way to ensure a successful outcome for all. It is not your job to take care of global problems, but your increased awareness of them may provide added incentive to make a difference in your own home. I hope the lessons in this book will help you to maintain perspective and to pass along the essential lessons to build body esteem in your children.

THE TEN ESSENTIAL LESSONS, IN REVIEW

For body esteem and health, begin by accepting what is *not* in your control:

1. Accept your body's genetic predisposition. All bodies are wired to be fatter, thinner, or in-between. This includes fatter in some places and thinner in others. Regardless of efforts to change it, your body will fight to maintain or

resume the overall shape it was born to be. You may temporarily force your body into a size that you prefer, but you can't beat Mother Nature without a tremendous cost.

2. Understand that bodies change developmentally in ways that are simply not in your control through healthy means. You may have a positive *influence* on changes in appearance occurring with puberty, pregnancy and lactation, menopause, and aging by making healthy lifestyle choices, but you will not "control" these changes, no matter how much you try.

3. Never diet. Hunger is an internally regulated drive and demands to be satisfied. If you limit the amount and quality of food needed to satiate hunger in hopes of losing weight, it will backfire, triggering preoccupation with food and ultimately an overeating or compulsive eating response. You may lose weight in the short run, but 95 percent of weight that is lost through dieting is regained, often with additional pounds. Dieters who go off their diets by bingeing are not "weak willed." They are mammals whose built-in starvation response has kicked in—both physically and psychologically—going after what has been restricted. Scientific evidence has been available on this since the early 1950s, but most people are still not aware of the biologically predictable counterproductive results of dieting.

Next, focus your attention and energy on what *is* within your control to achieve success and feel good:

4. Satisfy hunger completely with plenty of wholesome, nutrient-rich foods chosen from the core of the food pyra-

mid—*eat well!* Once your hunger is satiated, you will find it much easier to limit high-fat, low-nutrient "entertainment" snacks.

5. Limit sedentary entertainment. Move aerobically on a regular basis, if possible. Just about everyone, regardless of size, can and should develop a reasonable level of fitness.

6. Understand that if you eat well and maintain an active lifestyle over time, your best, natural weight will be revealed. Decide to eat well and be active. Don't be swayed by whether or not this makes you thin. Healthy, well-fed, active bodies are diverse in size and shape, from fat to thin and everything in between. Don't let anyone tell you otherwise, not even medical personnel, who may still be caught in unhealthy cultural myths about weight.

7. Choose role models who reflect a realistic standard against which you can feel good about yourself. If the "ugly duckling" had continued to compare herself to the ducks, she'd *still* be miserable, no matter how beautifully she developed.

8. Maintain your integrity as a human being. In spite of seductive advertisements that encourage you to believe "image is everything," never forget that how you look is only one part of who you are. Develop your sense of identity based on all the many things you can do and the person that you are deep inside.

9. Become media savvy. Educate yourself about the hidden power of advertisements. Advertisers spend tons of money on strategies specifically designed to make you feel that there is something wrong with you. Why? If you didn't

feel deficient, why else would you buy their products? Don't be "sold" this bill of goods.

10. Encourage your friends to join you in developing a healthy, realistic body image and challenging the status quo. Use all the collective energy you might otherwise have spent hating your bodies for a better cause.

APPENDIX A

BODY IMAGE AND
EATING CONTINUUM

Which level best describes your body image and approach to eating?

PHASE ONE
Level 1-A: No concerns. You have a very healthy body image and approach to eating.
- You generally accept your body. You might *prefer* to have different body characteristics that would give you a different look, but you understand the limits of your genetically predisposed body.
- You strongly value good physical health and emotional well-being, and make choices based on this.
- You trust your body to regulate your weight, and you satisfy hunger with a wide variety of wholesome foods. You enjoy exercise and physical activity for fun and fitness. You balance entertainment eating with a return to healthy eating. You never diet, regardless of your weight.
- You choose realistic role models against whom you feel good about yourself.

Level 1-B: You have a few minor concerns, but do not allow these to interfere with healthy choices.

- You may look longingly at role models who perpetuate the "thin ideal," but maintain your perspective.

- You feel some dissatisfaction with certain aspects of your size and shape, but this is held in check by acceptance of your biological inheritance.

- You feel tempted by the promise of dieting in hopes of more closely approximating the "thin ideal," but understand dieting is a self-defeating choice. You know that healthy options include eating well, staying physically fit, and making the most of the body size and shape that results.

PHASE TWO

Level 2-A: You have some clear body image and eating concerns.

- You are dissatisfied with your body and want to resist the limits of your genetic predisposition. You "feel fat" or that parts are "fat" (negative connotation implied) regardless of size, and you want to "do something" about it.

- You value health and well-being, but will deny your nutritional needs and hunger at times in hopes this will result in weight loss.

- You begin to periodically diet or restrict eating, hoping to lose weight. You are mentally preoccupied with eating and not eating. You begin to think of exercise as a way to burn calories.

- You routinely compare yourself to role models chosen primarily for their desired looks.

Level 2-B: You meet or nearly meet the minimum criteria for a borderline eating disorder. You may need professional help to regain a healthy perspective and healthy lifestyle.

- You are preoccupied most days with negative judgments and self-talk about your body. You are disgusted by your real or perceived body fat. You devote time to weighing, measuring, posturing, and scrutinizing your body.

- You are continuously thinking about plans to lose weight through whatever means may work. You are willing to sacrifice health and significant daily time to this cause in hopes of losing weight (or maintaining a low weight).

- You expend considerable energy denying hunger through restrictive eating. You may experience compulsive or binge-eating episodes following restrictive periods. These renew the desire to begin the diet cycle again.

- You blame yourself rather than observing that dieting is counterproductive (i.e., that dieting increases obsession with and loss of control over food). You may engage in more dangerous purging on occasion. You may exercise compulsively to burn calories.

- You are very preoccupied with the belief that weight loss is essential to desirability.

PHASE THREE

Level 3-A: You have a diagnosable eating disorder. Professional treatment is indicated.

- You are consumed with disdain for your body. You objectify and feel cut off from your body. Severe all-or-nothing self-judgments vary but depend on very small changes in weight (e.g., fat/ugly/gross versus thin/OK/relief) with very little ground between. You may have an extremely distorted view of your body size.

- You are obsessed with the activities involved in rigid restriction and regulation of eating and have little or no regard for nutritional needs. Your obsessive thoughts and compulsive behaviors are no longer within your control and take over most of your daily waking hours.
- Extreme weight loss efforts may alternate with uncontrollable compulsive and binge eating. You routinely engage in purging behaviors: starvation, vomiting, laxative use, or other means designed to eliminate food or avoid it.
- You may engage in a rigid, uncompromising exercise regime that can consume several hours per day.
- Weight may or may not fall to a level that is a danger to life, but your behavior seriously compromises health. You deny the problem and go to great lengths to maintain this facade. You may admit the problem, but are unable to consider healthy alternatives due to delusional ideation about controlling weight.

Level 3-B: Your eating disorder is life threatening.

- Your eating disorder has progressed to the point that you are medically unstable. Hospitalization is essential.

A one-page printable version of this continuum is available at www.bodyimagehealth.org.

APPENDIX B

THE MODEL FOR HEALTHY BODY IMAGE©
Developed by Kathy J. Kater, LICSW

Conceptual Building Blocks	Foundation	Desired Outcome	Goal
Developmental change is inevitable. Normal changes of puberty include weight gain and temporary out-of-proportion growth; <u>fat</u> does not define "overweight." Genetics and other internal weight regulators limit the degree to which shape, weight, and BMI can be manipulated through healthy means. Restricted or restrained hunger results in predictable consequences that are <u>counterproductive</u> to weight loss and interfere with normal hunger regulation.	Respect basic biology; understand what cannot be controlled about size, shape, and hunger	Acceptance of the innate body: "This is the body I was born to have."	**Healthy Body Image**
Balance attention to <u>many</u> aspects of identity. Looks are only one part. Satisfy hunger with <u>enough</u> varied, wholesome food in a stable, consistent manner. Limit sedentary choices to promote a physically active lifestyle. Choose role models who reflect a realistic standard.	Emphasize what <u>can</u> be influenced or chosen	Eating well for satisfaction of hunger, nutrition, and enjoyment (<u>not</u> "to lose weight"). Limited eating purely for "entertainment." A physically active lifestyle for fitness, fun, relaxation, and stress relief (<u>not</u> "to lose weight"). Limited sedentary entertainment.	**Prevention of Unhealthy and Disordered Eating**
Promote historical perspective on cultural attitudes related to body image. Teach and encourage critical thinking regarding media messages that influence body image. Support others in resisting unhealthy social norms about weight, dieting, low-nutrient food choices, and sedentary entertainment.	Develop social and cultural resiliency	Autonomy, self-esteem, confidence, and the ability for critical thinking.	

THE BUILDING BLOCKS FOR HEALTHY BODY IMAGE

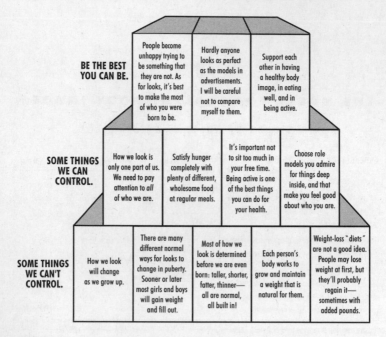

BE THE BEST YOU CAN BE.

People become unhappy trying to be something that they are not. As for looks, it's best to make the most of who you were born to be.

Hardly anyone looks as perfect as the models in advertisements. I will be careful not to compare myself to them.

Support each other in having a healthy body image, in eating well, and in being active.

SOME THINGS WE CAN CONTROL.

How we look is only one part of us. We need to pay attention to *all* of who we are.

Satisfy hunger completely with plenty of different, wholesome food at regular meals.

It's important not to sit too much in your free time. Being active is one of the best things you can do for your health.

Choose role models you admire for things deep inside, and that make you feel good about who you are.

SOME THINGS WE CAN'T CONTROL.

How we look will change as we grow up.

There are many different normal ways for looks to change in puberty. Sooner or later most girls and boys will gain weight and fill out.

Most of how we look is determined before we are even born: taller, shorter, fatter, thinner— all are normal, all built in!

Each person's body works to grow and maintain a weight that is natural for them.

Weight-loss "diets" are not a good idea. People may lose weight at first, but they'll probably regain it— sometimes with added pounds.

From the Model for Healthy Body Image by Kathy J. Kater, LICSW © 1998–2001 BodyImageHealth.org

APPENDIX C

DO YOU EAT ENOUGH?

Cheryl's Story

The graphs on pages 239 and 240 were completed by Cheryl, a thirty-six-year-old woman who had asked for help with her "overeating." Cheryl told me that she ate way too much every day. She wanted to overcome her lack of willpower when it came to eating, to eat normally so that she would stop hating herself for being "such a pig" and to lose weight. I include samples of Cheryl's "Do You Eat Enough?" pages because her problems typify those of so many children and adults who have eating problems. Cheryl's weight doesn't matter, because I have heard variations of her story from women who were size 0 to size 24, and ages eleven to sixty-five.

Listening to Cheryl, I learned that in grade school she had been a slim, athletic child who had always amazed her moderately plump family by the amount of food she could eat and still remain slender. In particular, she never passed on sweets and would eat them whenever she had the chance. Cheryl developed a little late compared to her friends, but began to round out in the seventh grade, when she gained both height and weight, and became a little "pudgy" (her word).

At that time her mother and aunts, who were always comparing diets, began to remark to her that she had better "watch it" or she would end up fat, like them. She began her first diet at age fourteen and had not stopped cycling on and off some diet plan or other since that time.

After reaching her full height in eighth grade (when she began dieting), Cheryl's weight had remained within the same ten-pound range for eighteen years. Cheryl was sure the slender body of her childhood had been trapped inside her fat, "ugly" body all that time. She had maintained her involvement in physical activity through the years and was engaged in some form of intense exercise almost daily: biking, running, tennis, racket ball, running, skiing, aerobic walking—you name it, she did it. She was sure it was her "overeating" that was the problem for the pounds she hated.

Like many people I work with, I told Cheryl I was frankly worried that she might not be eating enough. After first doubting my credibility and then my sanity, she assured me that once I heard all she could pack away in a day, I would have no doubt that it was "too much food." I sent her home with the "Do You Eat Enough?" worksheets, and a week later she brought back seven pages of eating records, but no graph. She had felt too ashamed to log the results. It was one thing to tell me in general that she "overate," but another to actually show me the quantity of food she had consumed.

We plotted the graph together in my office, with her reading the number of servings, while I marked the paper. When we had finished I handed the results, shown on page 239, back to her. "So what do you think? Do you eat enough?" She automatically started to roll her eyes, indicating the answer was obviously, "More than enough!" but I stopped her, insisting she actually look at the paper in front of her.

"Did you eat enough grain?"
Cheryl: "Uh, I guess not."

"Did you eat enough vegetables?"
Cheryl: "Well, no."

"Fruit?"
Cheryl: "Well, on two days I did."

"How about dairy?"
Cheryl: "Most days."

"Did you eat enough protein?"
Cheryl: "Uh, about half the time."

"Was this a typical week for you?"
Cheryl: "I think so."

"So, do you eat enough?"
Cheryl (starting to cry): "But look at all the junk I ate!"

"Well, yes I see that you ate your share of 'junk.' But did you eat enough of what your body needs?"
Cheryl (crying hard now and shaking her head): "No. But what about all the junk?"

"Honestly Cheryl, I think it's putting the cart before the horse to worry about the treats you eat. First, I think we need to find out what would happen if you would be willing to eat enough of what your body needs for a change. Once you are doing that, if you are still eating this many high-fat/sugar foods, we can talk about it. But until then, I think we'd better see if we can help

you to eat enough of the nutrients you need. Can you tell me why you're crying, Cheryl?"

Cheryl: "I always loved to eat as a kid, but ever since I was in seventh grade, people have been telling me I eat too much. No one has ever told me I don't eat enough. I can't believe it. It's just overwhelming!"

I sent Cheryl home with more "Do You Eat Enough?" pages, telling her not to worry about how much junk food she ate, but that her goal should be to try to eat enough servings of foods from all the other food groups. When she returned, she brought the already-completed graph on page 240. After eighteen years of trying to limit her sweet tooth through willpower and restriction, Cheryl found that the best control was her own internal hunger regulation. When she ate enough of the wholesome foods her body needed, she still enjoyed her sweet tooth, but was amazed to find she had much less interest in and room for all the treats she was so accustomed to craving.

The eating transformation made by Cheryl is admittedly remarkable for someone with years of restrictive and negligent eating behind her. It is rarely so easy. My wish is that we teach our children the lessons that Cheryl learned about healthy eating and body image so that they might avoid years of struggle and unhappiness.

DO YOU EAT ENOUGH? WEEKLY GRAPH

- Mark the number of servings you ate each day from each food group.
- Reach to the gray for the minimum each day!

1. Do you eat enough from each food group?   2. If not, how can you make room for what you need?

Servings per day of grains

Day	1	2	3	4	5	6	7	8	9	10	11	12
1												
2												
3												
4												
5												
6												
7												

Servings per day of vegetables

Day	1	2	3	4	5	6	7	8	9	10	11	12
1												
2												
3												
4												
5												
6												
7												

Servings per day of fruits

Day	1	2	3	4	5	6	7	8	9	10	11	12
1												
2												
3												
4												
5												
6												
7												

Servings per day of protein

Day	1	2	3	4	5	6	7	8	9	10	11	12
1												
2												
3												
4												
5												
6												
7												

Servings per day of dairy

Day	1	2	3	4	5	6	7	8	9	10	11	12
1												
2												
3												
4												
5												
6												
7												

Servings per day of fats and sweets

Day	1	2	3	4	5	6	7	8	9	10	11	12
1												
2												
3												
4												
5												
6												
7												

Cheryl's Results week 2
DO YOU EAT ENOUGH? WEEKLY GRAPH

- Mark the number of servings you ate each day from each food group.
- Reach to the gray for the minimum each day!

1. Do you eat enough from each food group?   **2. If not, how can you make room for what you need?**

Servings per day of grains

Day	1	2	3	4	5	6	7	8	9	10	11	12

Servings per day of vegetables

Day	1	2	3	4	5	6	7	8	9	10	11	12

Servings per day of fruits

Day	1	2	3	4	5	6	7	8	9	10	11	12

Servings per day of protein

Day	1	2	3	4	5	6	7	8	9	10	11	12

Servings per day of dairy

Day	1	2	3	4	5	6	7	8	9	10	11	12

Servings per day of fats and sweets

Day	1	2	3	4	5	6	7	8	9	10	11	12

APPENDIX D

RECOMMENDED READING, REFERENCES, AND RESOURCES

Innumerable books offer the "latest/greatest weight loss plan," or advice on how to help anyone be "thin for life." Most of these books contribute to our culture's body-image, eating, and weight problems. An additional, smaller group of books contain sound information about eating and activity, but are not recommended here because their underlying premise is that *any* child who achieves a healthy lifestyle will lose weight and/or be slim. Even if this prophesy holds true for many children, since it does not hold true for *all*, such books perpetuate destructive myths that deny the limits to our control over weight. In contrast, the following books and resources contain sound information that does not contradict what we know is true about healthy eating, fitness, and weight for everyone, regardless of size or predisposition.

Feeding Children

Child of Mine: Feeding with Love and Good Sense by Ellyn Satter (Bull Publishing, 2000).

How to Get Your Kids to Eat, But Not Too Much by Ellyn Satter (Bull Publishing, 1987).

How to Teach Nutrition to Kids by Connie Liakos Evers (24 Carrot Press, 2003).

Intuitive Eating by Evelyn Tribole (St. Martin's Press, 1996).

The Mom's Guide to Meal Makeovers by Janice Bissex and Liz Weiss (Broadway Books, 2004).

The Secrets of Feeding a Healthy Family by Ellyn Satter (Kelcy Press, 1999).

Fitness

The Bodywise Woman by Judy Lutter and Lynn Jaffee (Human Kinetics, 1996).

365 Activities for Fitness, Fun and Food for the Whole Family by Julia Sweet and Michael Jacobson (McGraw Hill Contemporary Books, 2001).

Promoting Healthy Weight Attitudes in Boys and Girls

Preventing Childhood Eating Problems: A Practical, Positive Approach for Raising Children Free of Food and Weight Conflicts by Jane Hirschman and Lela Zaphiropoulos (Gurze Books, 1993).

Promoting Healthy Weight Attitudes for Girls

Body Thieves by Sandra Friedman (Salal Books, 2002).

Dads and Daughters by Joe Kelly (Broadway Books, 2002).

Girls Will Be Girls: Raising Confident and Courageous

Daughters by JoAnn Deak, Ph.D., and Teresa Barker (Hyperion, 2002).

Like Mother, Like Daughter: How Girls and Women Are Influenced by Their Mother's Relationship with Food and How to Break the Pattern by Debra Waterhouse (Hyperion, 1997).

Over It: A Teens Guide to Getting Beyond Obsession with Food and Weight by Carol Emery Normandi and Laurelee Roark (New World Library, 2001).

Raising a Healthy Daughter: Parents and the Awakening of a Healthy Woman by Jeanne Elium and Don Elium (Celestial Arts Publishing, 2003).

Reviving Ophelia: Saving the Selves of Adolescent Girls by Mary Pipher (Ballantine Books, 2002).

Schoolgirls: Young Women, Self-Esteem, and the Confidence Gap by Peggy Orenstein (Doubleday, 1994).

Seven Strategies for Growing a Girl by Barbara Mackoff, Ph.D. (Dell, 1996).

200 Ways to Raise a Girl's Self-Esteem by Will Glennon (Conari Press, 1999).

Urban Girls: Resisting Stereotypes, Creating Identities edited by Bonnie J. Ross Leadbeater and Niobe Way (New York University Press, 1996).

When Girls Feel Fat: Helping Girls Through Adolescence by Sandra Friedman (Firefly Books, 2000).

You Have to Say I'm Pretty, You're My Mother: How to Help Your Daughter Learn to Love Her Body and Herself by Stephanie Pierson and Phyllis Cohen (Simon and Schuster, 2003).

Concerns of Boys and Men

The Adonis Complex: The Secret Crisis of Male Body Obsession by Harrison Pope Jr., Katherine Phillips, Robert Olivardia (Free Press, 2000).

Boys Will Be Boys: Breaking the Link Between Masculinity and Violence by Miriam Miedzian (Anchor Books, 1991).

Looking Good: Male Body Image in America by Lynne Luciano (Hill & Wang, 2002).

Making Weight: Healing Men's Conflicts with Food, Weight and Shape by Arnold Andersen, Leigh Cohn, Tom Holbrook, and Thomas M. Holbrook (Gurze Books, 2000).

Real Boys: Rescuing Our Sons from the Myths of Boyhood by William Pollack (Random House, 1998).

Causes of Body-Image, Weight, and Eating Problems

Afraid to Eat: Children and Teens in Weight Crisis by Frances Berg (Healthy Weight Network, 1997).

Appetites: Why Women Want by Caroline Knapp (Counterpoint/Perseus Books Group, 2003).

The Beauty Myth: How Images of Beauty Are Used Against Women by Naomi Wolf (Perennial, 2002).

Big Fat Lies: The Truth About Your Weight and Your Health by Glenn Gaessner (Gurze Books, 2002).

Bodylove: Learning to Like Our Looks and Ourselves: A Practical Guide for Women by Rita Freeman (Gurze Books, 2002).

The Body Project: An Intimate History of American Girls by Joan Jacobs Brumberg (Vintage, 1998).

Eating Problems: A Feminist Psychoanalytic Treatment Model by Carol Bloom (Basic Books, 1994).

Fasting Girls: The Emergence of Anorexia Nervosa as a Modern Disease by Joan Blumberg (Vintage, 2002).

Fat History: Bodies and Beauty in the Modern West by Peter N. Stearns (New York University Press, 1999).

Fat Is a Feminist Issue by Susie Orbach (Budget Book Service, 1997).

A Hunger So Wide and Deep: A Multicultural View of Women's Eating Problems by Becky Thompson (University of Minnesota Press, 1996).

The Hungry Self: Women, Eating and Identity by Kim Chernin, (Perennial Press, 1994).

The Invisible Woman: Confronting Weight Prejudice in America by W. Charisse Goodman (Gurze Books, 1995).

Just the Weigh You Are by Linda Konner and Steven Jonas (Houghton-Mifflin, 1998).

Life Inside the Thin Cage: A Personal Look Inside the Life of a Chronic Dieter by Constance Rhodes (Shaw, 2003).

Losing It: False Hopes and Fat Profits in the Diet Industry by Laura Fraser (Penguin Books, 1998).

The Obsession: Reflections on the Tyranny of Slenderness by Kim Chernin (Perennial Press, 1994).

Real Gorgeous: The Truth about Bodies and Beauty by Kaz Cooke (Norton, 1995).

The Skinny on Fat by Shawna Vogel (W. H. Freeman & Company, 1999).

True Beauty: Positive Attitudes and Practical Tips from the World's Leading Plus-Sized Model by Emme (Perigee, 1998).

Unbearable Weight: Feminism, Western Culture, and the Body by Susan Bordo (Unversity of California Press, 1995).

Underage and Overweight: America's Childhood Obesity Epidemic by Frances Berg (Hatherleigh Press, 2004).

When Women Stop Hating Their Bodies by Jane Hirshman and Carol Munter (Ballantine Books, 1996).

Professional, Academic, and Research Texts

Body Image, Eating Disorders, and Obesity: An Integrative Guide for Assessment and Treatment edited by J. Kevin Thompson (American Psychological Association, 1996).

Body Image, Eating Disorders, and Obesity in Youth: Assessment Prevention and Treatment by J. Kevin Thompson and Linda Smolak (American Psychological Association, 2001).

Body Image: A Handbook of Research, Theory and Clinical Practice by Thomas Cash and Thomas Pruzinsky (Guilford Press, 2002).

Child and Adolescent Obesity: Causes and Consequences, Prevention and Management edited by Thomas Wadden and Albert Stunkard (Cambridge University Press, 2002).

The Developmental Psychopathology of Eating Disorders: Implications for Research, Prevention and Treatment edited by Linda Smolak, Michael P. Levine, Ruth Striegel-Moore (Lawrence Erlbaum Associates, 1996).

Eating Disorders: Obesity, Anorexia Nervosa and the Person Within by Hilda Bruch (Basic Books, 1985).

Exacting Beauty: Theory, Assessment, and Treatment of Body Image Disturbance by J. Thompson (American Psychological Association, 1999).

Interpreting Weight: The Social Management of Fatness and Thinness by Jeffery Sobal and Donna Maurer (Aldine de Gruyter, 1999).

Moving Away from Diets by Karin Kratina, Nancy King, and
Dale Hayes (Helm Publishing, 2003).

*Preventing Eating Disorders: A Handbook of Interventions
and Special Challenges* by Niva Piran, Michael P. Levine,
and Catherine Steiner-Adair (Brunner-Routledge, 1999).

Understanding Eating Disorders edited by Alexander Lumsden and D. Lumsden (Taylor & Francis, 1994).

Eating Disorders

Anatomy of Anorexia by Steven Levenkron (W. W. Norton &
Company, 2001).

*Consuming Passions: Feminist Approaches to Weight Preoccu-
pation and Eating Disorders* edited by Catrina Brown and
Karin Jasper (Second Story Press, 1994).

*Dying to Be Thin: Understanding and Defeating Anorexia
Nervosa and Bulimia* by Ira Sacker and Marc Zimmer
(Warner Books, 2001).

*The Eating Disorder Sourcebook: A Comprehensive Guide to
the Causes, Treatment and Prevention of Eating Disorders*
by Carolyn Costin (McGraw-Hill/Contemporary Books,
1999).

*Helping Your Child Overcome an Eating Disorder: What You
Can Do at Home* by Bethany Teachman (editor) (New
Harbinger Publishers, 2003).

Hunger Pains: From Fad Diets to Eating Disorders by Mary
Pipher (Ballantine Books, 1997).

Your Dieting Daughter: Is She Starving for Attention by Carolyn Costin (Brunner/Mazel Trade, 1996).

*When Your Child Has an Eating Disorder: A Step-by-Step
Workbook for Parents and Other Caregivers* by Abigail
Natenshon (Jossey-Bass, 1999).

Stories by or about Eating Disorder Sufferers

The Best Little Girl in the World by Steven Levenkron (Warner Books, 1989).

Room to Grow: An Appetite for Life by Tracey Gold (New Millennium Press, 2003).

Stick Figure: A Diary of My Former Self by Lori Gottlieb (Berkely Publishing Group, 2001).

Wasted: A Memoir of Anorexia and Bulimia by Marya Hornbacher (HarperCollins, 1999).

Books for Children

Pre-school and older

The Edible Pyramid: Good Eating Every Day by Loreen Leedy (Scott Foresman Publishing, 1996).

I Like Me by Nancy Carlson (Viking, 1988).

I Love My Hair by Natasha Anastasia Tarpley (Little, Brown, 1998).

Shapesville by Andy Mills and Becky Osborn (Gurze Books, 2003).

The Straight Line Wonder by Mem Fox (Mondo Publishing, 1997).

Wings by Christopher Myers (Scholastic Press, 2000).

Ages seven and older

Albertina the Practically Perfect by Susi Gregg Fowler (Greenwillow, 1998).

Because of Winn-Dixie by Kate DiCamillo (Candlewick Press, 2000).

Stephanie's Ponytail by Robert Munsch (Annick Press, 1996).

When the Circus Came to Town by Laurence Yep (Harper-Collins, 2002).

Ages ten and older

Blubber by Judy Blume (Yearling Books, 1976).

Body Talk: Straight Facts about Fitness, Nutrition, and Feeling Great about Yourself! by Ann and Julie Douglas (Maple Tree Press, 2002).

Food and Nutrition for Every Kid by Janice Van Cleave (John Wiley and Sons, 1999).

Food Rules: The Stuff You Munch, Its Crunch, Its Punch, and Why You Sometimes Lose Your Lunch by Bill Haduch (Puffin, 2001).

Girl Power in the Mirror: A Book About Girls, Their Bodies, and Themselves by Helen Cordes (Lerner Publications Company, 1999).

The Healthy Body Cookbook: Over 50 Fun Activities and Delicious Recipes for Kids by Joan D'Amico (John Wiley and Sons, 1999).

Nell's Quilt by Susan Terris (Sunburst, 1996).

The Right Moves: A Girl's Guide to Getting Fit and Feeling Good by Tina Schwager and Michelle Shuerger (Free Spirit Publishing, 1998).

The Secret Life of Amanda K. Woods by Ann Cameron (Frances Foster Books/Farrar, Straus and Giroux, 1998).

The Sisterhood of the Traveling Pants by Ann Brashares (Delacorte Press, 2001).

Sisters/Hermanas by Gary Paulsen (Harcourt Brace & Company, 1993). Full text in Spanish and English.

Stay True: Short Stories for Strong Girls edited by Marilyn Singer (Scholastic Press, 1998).

The What's Happening to My Body Book for Boys by Linda
  Madaras (Newmarket Press, 2000).
The What's Happening to My Body Book for Girls by Linda
  Madaras (Newmarket Press, 2000).

Magazines for Girls

New Moon: The Magazine for Girls and Their Dreams, New
  Moon Publishing Phone: (800) 381–4743. Web site:
  www.newmoon.org.

Web Sites and Other Resources

BodyImageHealth.org. Information and resources by Kathy
  Kater.
Bodywise Information Packet, National Women's Health In-
  formation Center. Web site: www.4woman.gov/Body
  Image/Bodywise/bodywise.htm. Provides eating disorder resources for school personnel.
Get Moving for the Fun and Health of It., USDA Center
  for Nutrition Policy and Promotion. Web site: www
  .usda.gov/cnpp/Pubs/Brochures/index.html#Moving.
Kids in Action: Fitness for Children, Presidents Council on
  Physical Fitness and Kellogg's Company, 1996. Phone:
  (800) 822–0221.
Mind on the Media. Inspiring independent thinking and fos-
  tering critical analysis of media messages. This nonprofit
  is now the sponsor of Turn Beauty Inside Out Day. Web
  site: www.motm.org.
Parent's Guide to Physical Play, USDA Bureau of Nutrition
  & WIC. Phone: (800) 532–1579.
Physical Activity and Health: A Report of the Surgeon Gen-

eral, National Center for Disease Control. Web site: www.cdc.gov/nccdphp/sgr/prerep.htm.

USDA Food Guide Pyramid for Young Children, Tips for Using the Food Guide Pyramid with Children, USDA Center for Nutrition Policy and Promotion. Web site: www.usda.gov/cnpp.

Resources, Books, and Programs for Action

About Face. Web site: www.about-face.org. Promotes activism, healthy body image, and self-esteem in girls.

Body Wars: Making Peace with Women's Bodies, An Activist's Guide by Margo Maine (Gurze Books, 2000). Great information and resources for activism countering unhealthy cultural messages.

The Center for Media Literacy, 4724 Wiltshire Blvd., Suite 403, Los Angeles, CA 90010. Phone: (213) 931–4177. Web site: www.medialit.org. Provides resources on the impact of media influences.

Dads and Daughters, 32 East Superior Street, Suite 200, Duluth, MN 55802. Phone: (888) 824–3237. Web site: www.dadsanddaughters.org. Offers information, newsletters, forums and opportunities for activism to help dads inspire, understand, and support their daughters.

Girls on the Run: Box 268, Huntsville, NC 28070. Phone: (800) 901–9965. Web site: www.girlsontherun.com. Twelve-week program combining training for a 3.1-mile run with self-esteem-enhancing projects.

Gurze Books, Box 2238, Carlsbad, CA 92018. Phone: (800) 756–7553. Web site: www.gurze.com. Complete listing of books on eating disorders, free catalogue.

Just for Girls by Sandra Susan Friedman (Salal Books,

1999). Contains plans and handouts for group discussion.

MediaWatch (U.S.), P.O. Box 618, Santa Cruz, CA 95061–0618. Phone: (408) 423–6355. Web site: www.mediawatch.org. Dedicated to attacking sexism in advertising.

MediaWatch (Canada), 517 Wellington St. West, Suite 204, Toronto, ON M5V 1G1. Phone: (416) 408–2065. Web site: www.mediawatch.ca. Media watchdog, supports letter-writing campaigns.

Melpomene Institute for Women's Health Research, St. Paul, MN. Phone: (651) 642–1951. Web site: www.melpomene. org. Helps girls and women link physical activity and health through research, publications, and education.

National Eating Disorders Association, 603 Steward Street, Suite 803, Seattle WA 98101. Phone: (206) 382–3587. Web site: www.nationaleatingdisorders.org.

Something Fishy. Web site: www.somethingfishy.org. Provides solid information and resources related to eating disorders, as well as treatment referrals across the nation.

TV Turnoff Network. Web site: www.tvturnoff.org.

Curriculum

Am I Fat? Helping Young Children Accept Differences in Body Size by Joanne Ikeda and Priscilla Naworski (ETR Associates, 1993). Discussion guide for early grade school children.

GO GIRLS™ Program, National Eating Disorders Association, 603 Steward Street, Suite 803, Seattle, WA 98101. Phone: (206) 382–3587. Web site: www.neda.org. Provides inspiration and direction for teen groups that want to challenge unhealthy media messages.

Healthy Body Image: Teaching Kids to Eat and Love Their Bodies Too! by Kathy Kater, National Eating Disorders Association, 603 Steward Street, Suite 803, Seattle WA 98101. Phone: (206) 382–3587. Web site: www.neda.org. Comprehensive curriculum for upper elementary school children for prevention of body image, eating, and weight concerns. Adaptable for any age.

How to Say It to Girls by Nancy Gruver (Penguin, 2004). A practical guide on communicating with girls on 100 different topics.

New Moves by Dianne Neumark-Sztainer, School of Public Health, University of Minnesota, 1300 South Second Street, Suite 300, Minneapolis, MN 55454. Phone: (612) 626–7103. School-based obesity prevention program for adolescent girls.

KATHY KATER, LICSW, is a psychotherapist who has treated body image, eating, and weight concerns for twenty-five years. Frustrated that progress in understanding these problems had not been matched by effective prevention, she authored *Healthy Body Image: Teaching Kids to Eat and Love Their Bodies Too!* when her own daughter was about to enter fourth grade. This comprehensive prevention curriculum, published in 1998 by the National Eating Disorder Association, was among the first of its kind to demonstrate significant, measurable improvement in weight-related attitudes among pubescent children. *Healthy Body Image* is recommended by the U.S. Department of Health, Office of Women's Health, in its *BodyWise* information packet for educators, and is used in many schools across the country. Kathy Kater lives in St. Paul, Minnesota, with her husband, Lincoln Fletcher, son, Adam, and daughter, Anya.

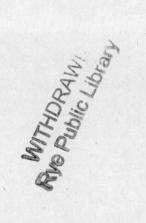